WELLNESS EQ PUBLISHI

CW00642549

EAT WELL OR DIE SLC...

'Eat Well or Die Slowly is a compelling short story challenging the misinformation surrounding "nutrition science". Estrelita and Issy weave us through the tangled web surrounding the vilification of saturated fats, highlighting the influence of vested interests pushing a nutrient deficient diet that is compromising our health. The easy conversational style, fun graphics and well referenced content make this an engaging educational book that may just be the beginning of your journey back to health.'

Belinda Fettke, Registered Nurse,
Co-Founder of Nutrition for Life,
Tasmania, Australia

'I really have to take my hat off to the authors of this book. They have neatly and clearly summarised the central research and concepts that are needed to convince people that a real food diet is the key to health and happiness. This will be a wonderful resource for people to learn how to heal metabolic health problems but also to educate families and even health practitioners to support those of us trying not to live according to the received (yet incorrect) dietary dogma of low fat and high carbohydrates. Optimal physical and mental health await!'

Dr Jen Unwin, UK Consultant Clinical Health
Psychologist and Member of the Public Health
Collaboration Scientific Advisory Board

Eat Well
or
Die Slowly

Eat Well or Die Slowly

GUIDE TO METABOLIC HEALTH

Dr Estrelita van Rensburg and Issy Warrack

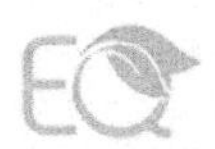

Published by Wellness EQ Publishing

The information in this book is provided to assist the reader in making informed choices about their diet. This book is not intended as a substitute for medical advice and anybody changing their diet should consult their physician about the treatment implications of any underlying medical conditions.

Figures designed by Estrelita van Rensburg

Cover design by Elisabeth Heissler Design

ISBN 978 1 8381378 0 9 (Paperback)

ISBN 978 1 8381378 1 6 (eBook)

Visit us at www.wellnesseq.net

ACKNOWLEDGEMENTS

We started writing this book at the start of the COVID-19 lockdown in the UK, having already carried out extensive research in the preceding eighteen months. We had also devised a low-carb eating Programme which we had successfully trialled and subsequently launched so were able to see the results for real and were sure we were on the right track.

We genuinely appreciate the part that our early participants played in this Programme. Their positive and constructive feedback was very welcome.

We gratefully acknowledge the following who, as well as providing support and encouragement, played an instrumental role in proofreading the original manuscript: Chrissie Bell, Professor Anne-Marie Beukes, Lizette Robbertze and Malcolm Warrack. In particular, we would like to thank Professor Johan Joubert, a microbiologist with considerable experience in biochemistry, for his helpful discussions on how to accurately describe complex biochemical processes to make it accessible to non-medical people.

I (Estrelita) wish to thank Issy for her encouragement in getting this project started, for being a sounding board for ideas and always willing to hunt down relevant information sources. My deep gratitude to my mother, Hettie, who always encouraged and supported me when I embarked on new projects.

I (Issy) wish to thank my co-author and partner Estrelita, whose original comment 'You'll have to change your diet', got me right back on track to leading a full healthy reenergised life. Her encouragement knows no bounds. I acknowledge too the role my daughter, Sally, has had in driving me personally forward to lead life to the full, appreciating every day. Life is for living.

CONTENTS

LIST OF FIGURES

INTRODUCTION

'The words of truth are simple.'

Aeschylus

We commenced writing this book at the start of the COVID-19 lockdown. It was an opportunity to start a big project because everything else had ground to a halt. At least the internet was not affected, so there was no problem accessing the required references and information. For me (Estrelita) it was a strange time. Here I was, a retired clinical virologist, who was no longer active in the field. It felt like I was sitting on the fence looking at the biggest lockdown the world has ever seen without having a role to play. To think that a simple virus can have such a global impact is truly mind-blowing.

After studying medicine, I became interested in virology during the first decade of the HIV pandemic which provided many collaboration opportunities to work with scientists attempting to develop a vaccine. The HIV vaccine target has still not been achieved even today and, personally, I don't think it ever will. But COVID-19 is a very different virus, and developing a vaccine is definitely doable and will be the most important tool to bring this pandemic under control.

COVID-19 brought to our attention the fact that there are certain subgroups of people who become severely ill with a much higher mortality rate than the rest of the affected population. People suffering from obesity, diabetes and heart disease are much more at risk of severe disease and complications. These lifestyle diseases are the tip of the iceberg of a much larger and more insidious pandemic that has been creeping up on us over the last 40 years and which is escalating in mega proportions, the likes of which the world has never seen before. This is the epidemic of diseases related to our modern-day diet of which most people, including the medical community, are not even aware.

Why am I writing about this? Since retiring from academia and the pharmaceutical industry, I have become increasingly interested in the prevention of disease. I knew that nutrition was important, but it was definitely not a topic that I was previously even vaguely interested in. I am sure that many of my medical colleagues feel the same. Were we not taught at medical school how important it was to diagnose disease and then taught which drugs to prescribe to treat our patient's symptoms? Nutrition was never high on the list and certainly something that most physicians are not, even today, comfortable discussing with their patients.

Getting back to my story, my idea was to quickly skim over the basics of nutrition and then move on to more interesting topics on how to live healthily. Or so I thought! What I discovered was initially unbelievable and then, further on, I was truly astounded by the magnitude of misinformation in this area. It shook the very foundations of what we were taught at medical school. The fact that mainstream media as well as the medical profession are supporting these false beliefs, advising the general population to participate in a nutrition programme that is utterly damaging to their health, makes me angry, to say the least. It is this deception and my own anger that has driven me ever since to help people understand the truth.

Because of my own research career, I am very familiar with reviewing scientific data and was therefore in no way daunted by the task of familiarising myself with my new field of interest: nutrition.

When you read this book, keep an open mind. Your beliefs, just as ours were, will be challenged! We have all come to believe that the older we get, our chances of getting sick with one or more chronic diseases are inevitable. It is just a fact of life and, when the time comes, we will get drugs from our GP to lower our blood pressure, lower our blood sugar, ease the pain in our weary joints and get a statin to lower our cholesterol, to mention just a few. It has become the new normal.

This reminds me of a conversation we had recently with a guy in his early sixties. When I asked if he suffered from any diseases, he assured me that he was healthy. When I asked if he was on any treatment, he said yes. He was on seven different medications for type 2 diabetes, high blood pressure and cholesterol. He thought that this was completely normal.

Why have we become so accepting of ill health being a normal condition? Is it perhaps because the older we get the more common it becomes to see family and friends suffering from one or more chronic conditions? Is ill health becoming synonymous with old age, a fate from which hardly anybody will escape? Recent surveys in the UK and US revealed that 42 to 49 per cent of adults today are concerned about developing Alzheimer's disease in their lifetime. This reminds me of the story of the 'boiling frog effect' – the notion that a frog immersed in gradually heated water will fail to notice the creeping change in its circumstances, even as it's literally being boiled alive. Are we ourselves all like frogs in the process of being boiled?

What if we tell you that by changing your diet you will be able to get rid of most of these fears and that it will result in powerful changes within your body to slow down, reverse or even put ongoing disease progression into remission. Too good to be true? Through our own experiences and those of many other people who have joined us or taken a similar journey, the results have been just exceptional. Stop and think for a moment about nature. Which wild animal living in their natural habitat suffers from chronic degenerative diseases (other than chronic infections)? We can't think of any, so why should it be different for humans? Prior to the era of modern medicine, say the last 100 years before the development of antibiotics, people died mainly of infectious diseases or injuries sustained during war or accidents, with chronic diseases very much in the background. This is in stark contrast to a recent report from the Centers for Disease Control and Prevention (CDC) that estimates 90 per cent of US national healthcare spending goes towards the management of chronic diseases and mental healthcare.

In this book, we will explore the surge of escalating chronic diseases in humans especially since the Second World War and the belief systems that were developed along the way based on bad science. The exploitation of these belief systems and bad science has led to extraordinary profits for the food, drink and pharmaceutical industries in the twentieth and twenty-first centuries. Big Business has just too much to lose to seriously review the scientific premise on which their products, advertising and lobbying campaigns are based. Governments, public health authorities and the whole of the medical profession are all engulfed in these beliefs.

They can't see the wood for the trees, because they are not allowed to or are unaware that there is another reality out there. Tactics employed to maintain the deception include perverse incentives such as research grants, funding of projects which always come with strings attached, sponsored trips with plush accommodation, disingenuous product advertising exploiting the unsuspecting medical fraternity and the vilification of anybody who dares to question the status quo.

Feeling sick already? Indeed, we hope so, because we need to sit up and take notice. The world is getting sicker and sicker, literally, while money is rolling into the big industries. Make up your own mind after reading this book. Help is, unfortunately, not going to come anytime soon from government or public health authorities – they have too much to lose. Losing face and funding at the same time is definitely too much to bear. Sad, but true.

In this book, we have tried to provide details of the history and some very complex and often confusing scientific discussions around the topic of nutrition. The aim is to present accurate, evidence-based data, without digging too deep into scientific jargon and intricate metabolic processes, in order to make the information accessible to anybody without a scientific or medical background. Once you understand the science behind good nutrition, you will be in a much better position to begin and experience the beginning of a life-changing journey. Some may say that we have left out a lot and simplified a very complex subject. To this we say, yes, we have focused on a few of the very important characters that played definitive and impactful roles whilst many others could have been included as well. But we do not think that it would have altered the message nor the science in any significant way.

Some scientific terminology is used, especially in Part 1, where we focus on the science and biology of nutrition. We hope that the explanations are adequate so that most people will feel comfortable with this section and understand the key points about how the choices we make regarding the food we eat can either keep us healthy or put us on a path to developing lifestyle diseases. In Part 2, we focus on food production since there has been such a massive change in farming methods and a meteoric rise in food manufacturing. This section begins with Issy's recollections of growing up on a farm in Scotland and how, in just two generations, the growing number of industrial farms have impacted the quality and quantity of the food we eat. The last chapter offers practical suggestions that will guide you on how to implement changes in your diet that will ignite a feel-good factor in your body – it certainly did for us! You will be amazed at how simple it really is. Now is the time to take responsibility for your own health. Bon voyage!

Part 1

BASIC SCIENCE OF FOOD AND DISEASE

Chapter 1

THE BASICS OF FOOD

'The greatest wealth is health.'

Virgil

Based on its chemical structure, food can be divided into macronutrients and micronutrients. There are three macronutrients: fat, protein and carbohydrates and two micronutrients: minerals and vitamins.

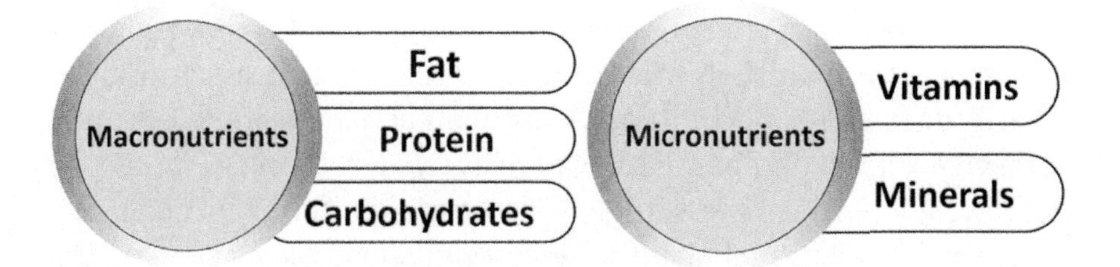

Figure 1. Macronutrients and micronutrients.

All of the micronutrients needed for physiological processes are found within the three macronutrients. In this discussion, we are going to concentrate on the macronutrient constituents. Only two of the three macronutrients are essential: fat and protein. In other words, we must eat these because without them our bodies cannot survive, and we will die. This means that we can survive without eating any carbohydrates. You may ask: *Really, what about all the vitamins, especially vitamin C?* Yes, indeed, all the required minerals and vitamins that we need, including vitamin C, are found in animal foods. For example, sufficient quantities of vitamin C are available in shellfish, chicken livers, veal and nuts.

Essential Macronutrients: Fat and Protein

Being healthy is all about eating food that is essential to support all the metabolic processes in our body. Current nutritional guidelines indicate that we should include all the different macronutrients in our diet. The guidelines instruct us to include a variety of colours and tastes, and ample portions of fruit and vegetables but, above all, advise us to be careful of fat and to make sure that we limit our intake of meat and other animal products.

We are going to explore this concept over the next few chapters and look at what evidence there is to support this view. We will also explore the consequences of following the current mainstream nutritional advice and see if it is in our best interest to pursue it.

One of the big questions regarding food is: Is it about *quantity* (i.e. calorie intake) or is it about *quality* (what we eat)? In answering this question, there are two main assumptions. The first assumption is that it doesn't so much matter what we eat – as long as we don't exceed a certain number of calories daily, we will be okay. Should we gain weight in the process, then it is a simple matter of cutting down our calorie intake, beefing up our willpower and joining a gym to burn off a few of those extra calories!

The second assumption is that calories don't matter – it is all about the type of foodstuffs we consume. If we do this correctly, our body's metabolism will keep us healthy and slim. I know which option I prefer – what about you? Let's explore the evidence and get to the heart of the matter.

We shall start by looking at the two essential macronutrients first: fat and protein.

Meet the Fat Family

Fat has been the most vilified macronutrient of the twentieth and twenty-first centuries, and we will look very closely at the reason for this later in the book.

There are different kinds of fat: those occurring naturally in food and those in man-made fats (made by the food industry). It is important to distinguish between the two because their chemical structures are different and the impact of the man-made or unnatural fats on our health is highly significant.

Fats (see Figure 2) are divided into saturated and unsaturated fats, with unsaturated fats divided into mono- and polyunsaturated fats.

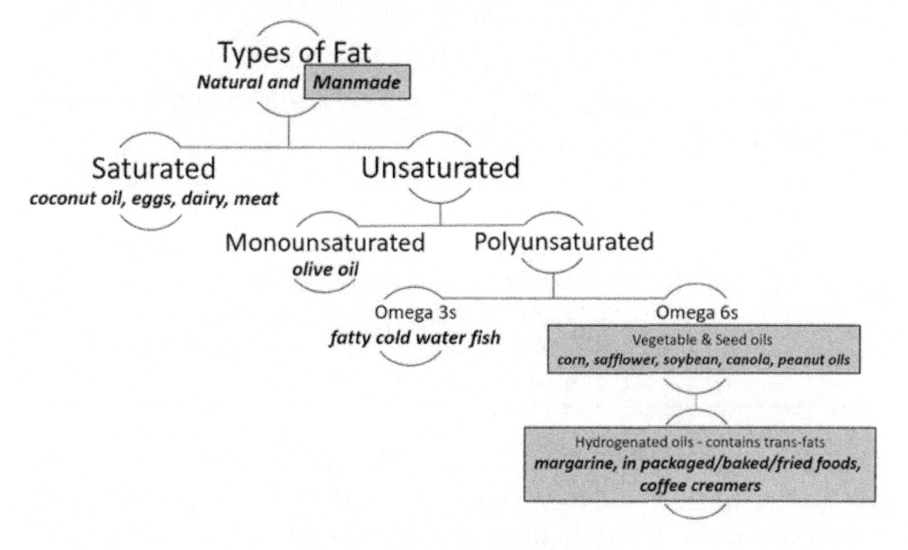

Figure 2. Classification of fats.

Scientists will point out that in biochemical terminology there is no such thing as a *fat* – it should be called a *fatty acid*. For those of you who are interested, a fatty acid is a string or backbone of carbon atoms linked to hydrogen atoms. One final bit of scientific information: the terms *saturated, unsaturated, mono-* and *poly*unsaturated refer to the number of double bonds in the fatty acid chain (the chain of carbon atoms). *Saturated* fats have no double bonds, while *un*saturated fats have one or more double bonds. In *mono*unsaturated fats, there is a single double bond while *poly*unsaturated fats have more than one double bond. Having explained all of that, to keep things simple, we are going to continue using the term *fat* when we refer to this macronutrient.

It is important to know that natural foods such as meat, fish, eggs and nuts contain all types of fats: saturated, monounsaturated and polyunsaturated fats. Dairy products are the only food group that contains more saturated than unsaturated fat, e.g. butter contains about 64 per cent saturated fat, while beef and lard contain only 40 per cent. Pork contains a higher amount of monounsaturated fat, similar to olive oil. It is interesting to note, contrary to popular belief that the highest amount of saturated fat content is not found in animal products, but in a plant: coconut oil, which contains 90 per cent saturated fat.

In order to make this fairly complicated subject clearer, we will use the term 'healthy fat' when we discuss fats naturally occurring in foods (see examples in the paragraph above)
while man-made, hydrogenated, vegetable
and/or seed oils all refer to processed or man-made fats
i.e. the 'unhealthy' group of fats.

Healthy fat has important functions in the body: it forms part of the membrane (protective wall) that surrounds every cell in our body, almost two-thirds of our brain is composed of fat and cholesterol, and our body uses fat as a fuel source, which is a much more efficient fuel source than carbohydrates. Fat is also the major storage form of energy in the body. Healthy fats are required to absorb the essential fat-soluble vitamins A, D, E and K from our gut (it is important to know that for effective absorption we need to eat full-fat products and not the 'low-fat' variety available in our supermarkets). Fat also makes food palatable and is satiating – keeping us full for longer!

Of all the fat-soluble vitamins, only vitamin E is naturally found in plant foods such as seeds (e.g. sunflower seeds) and nuts. Many plant foods are indeed rich in micronutrients, but just because a food type contains a particular nutrient doesn't necessarily mean it is the best available format of that nutrient which allows our body to absorb and utilise it efficiently. The scientific term for this is 'bioavailability'. For vitamins A, D and K, see the figure below for the types which have the highest bioavailability and therefore support our cellular functions best. Deficiency symptoms can develop if we (1) don't get enough of the correct nutrient, for example by avoiding animal foods, or (2) eat only low-fat products, which negatively impacts the absorption of fat-soluble vitamins.

Best Food Sources of Fat-Soluble Vitamins A, D and K

Vitamin	Main Functions	More potent type		Less potent type
A	brain: vision, learning, and memory; healthy skin & hair	Retinol liver, eggs, dairy	← *very low conversion rate*	Beta-carotene carrots, pumpkin
D	bone and tooth health	D_3 cholecalciferol oily fish, sunshine	← *inefficient conversion*	D_2 ergocalciferol sun-exposed mushrooms fortified foods
K	blood clotting & wound healing	K_2 (MK-4) liver, meat, cheese, eggs, fermented soy	← *inefficient & variable conversion*	K_1 leafy green vegetables

Figure 3. Best food sources of fat-soluble vitamins A, D and K.

Omega-3, one of the family of polyunsaturated fats has anti-inflammatory properties and is very important for brain development and intelligence. The best dietary source of omega-3 is fatty fish in your diet. Plant-based foods do not contain the correct type of omega-3 which our body needs and conversion of plant omega-3 (alpha-linolenic acid or ALA) to the types of omega-3 that we need (eicosapentaenoic acid or EPA and docosahexaenoic acid or DHA) is a very inefficient process. DHA is the most important omega-3 for our brain functions and makes up to 40 per cent of the total brain fat content.

In contrast, omega-6 is associated with inflammatory processes in the body. Its consumption has increased dramatically over the last century with the industrial production of vegetable and seed oils (see Figure 4).

History of Industrialised Polyunsaturated Fat Production

In *The Big Fat Surprise*, Nina Teicholz provides a detailed description of how industry started to create a completely new category of food in the nineteenth century and how, today, it is one of the most prevalent commodities used in processed food.

Up to the beginning of the twentieth century, housewives in Europe and North America used animal-origin fats. Oil was mainly used to make soaps, candles, waxes, lubricants and fuels. Oils made from seeds like cottonseeds were not considered acceptable for cooking and baking in the nineteenth century but, unbeknownst to consumers, manufacturers from the 1860s onwards started adding cottonseed oil to butter to reduce production costs. Mechanised processes for pressing cotton and other seeds (rape, safflower, sunflower, sesame), as well as corn and soybeans, became much more refined in the twentieth century, and these polyunsaturated oils became extremely popular for culinary use.

One downside of these unhealthy polyunsaturated fats was that they became rancid very quickly and that led to the hydrogenation process which rendered them solid depending on the amount of trans fats they contained. The more trans fats they contain the more solid they are. These alterations made them ideal for a whole myriad of uses by the processed food industry, such as chocolate coatings, cake icings, sauces, creamy fillings, and baking. In addition, they prolong the shelf life of the food and maintain flavour stability. Great news for the unsuspecting housewife since she now had products that would last forever!

From the 1960s onwards these new hydrogenated oils were even endorsed by the American Heart Association, which received millions of dollars in support from food companies who manufactured those oils. In 2011, Blasbalg et al. published a study on the consumption of fats in the US from 1909 to 1999 which estimated that the *per capita consumption of soybean oil increased >1000-fold from 1909 to 1999*.

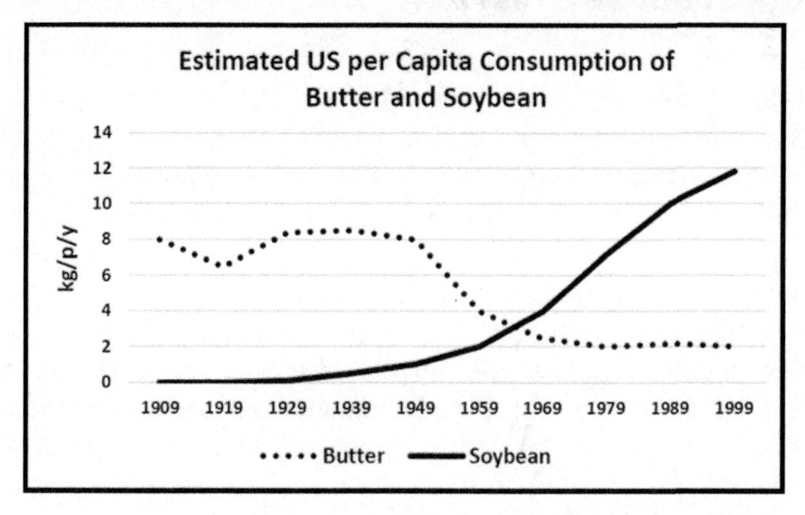

Figure 4. Changes in US per capita consumption of butter and soybean.

Redrawn from Blasbalg et al., *Am J Clin Nutr*, 2011.

This was achieved through aggressive and successful marketing campaigns by trade groups as well as recommendations to consume more polyunsaturated oils at the expense of animal fats. Since the beginning of the twentieth century, Americans have switched from eating animal fats to vegetable oils, especially soybean products, as can be seen in the butter vs soybean consumption graph (Figure 4).

Recent research has shown that an increase in omega-6 polyunsaturated fats is related to depression and mood disorders. Researchers think that this is because the traditional human diet supported an omega-3:omega-6 ratio of 1:1, while contemporary Western diets are characterised by a ratio of around 1:15 or higher, reflecting a deficient omega-3 intake and an excessive omega-6 intake through the consumption of processed food.

In addition, there are also reports of a possible link between exposure to the toxic residues from heated hydrogenated vegetable oils and the development of lung cancer in Chinese-style cooking.

More about Soy

Soy, a type of legume, contains many anti-nutrients that are not suitable for human consumption without a lot of processing. As seen in the previous section, soy as in soybean oil, is now the most commonly used vegetable oil and also a very important source of plant-based protein products (see below). Traditionally soy is found in the Asian diet and only eaten in small amounts in a fermented form (soy sauce, miso, tempeh, natto), which renders some of its toxic ingredients non-toxic. The British Committee on Toxicity (COT) reviewed data on possible detrimental effects of soy consumption in (1) soy-based infant formula and (2) the intake of soy-based food/soy dietary supplements and its impact on thyroid function. The conclusions from their Annual Reports are ambiguous and vague, e.g.:

- The 2013 COT Annual Report reviewed possible harmful effects of soy-based infant formula since it contains isoflavones that mimic the female hormone, oestrogen, and its potential impact on development and reproduction. They concluded that 'studies are too limited to provide strong reassurance of safety. Animal studies looking at similar levels of exposure to those reported in infants have suggested developmental and reproductive changes later in life'.

Not reassuring.

- With regard to soy's impact on hypothyroidism (underactive thyroid), the 2015 COT Annual Report states they don't think that soy 'impact(s) materially' on people with normal thyroid functions; however, it may precipitate symptoms in people with subclinical underactive thyroid disease or worsen the condition of people already on treatment, which could require them to increase their treatment dosage of thyroxine.

Again, not reassuring.

- In 2015 and 2020, researchers at the University of California, Riverside (Deol et al.) reported results of mice experiments which showed that soybean oil leads to obesity, diabetes, insulin resistance, fatty liver and also affects numerous genes influencing the brain's metabolism.

Even less reassuring.

Since the last two studies mentioned were conducted in mice, we cannot extrapolate these findings directly to humans. Nevertheless, it remains a concern which we should keep an eye on, especially in the face of several other concerns regarding anti-nutrients and toxins already identified in soy (see Figure 5).

Lierre Keith, in her book *The Vegetarian Myth*, mentions that soy-based infant formula contains, by a factor of several thousand, more isoflavones (compounds similar to the female hormone oestrogen) than human breast milk. The question mums should ask themselves is whether they want to expose their infants to such a high female hormonal load? Of further concern is that boys born with hypospadias (the opening of the urethra is on the underside of the penis rather than at the tip) are five times more likely to have a vegetarian mum.

Concerns about using Soy as a Food Source

Soy Effects: Anti-nutrient Properties	Symptoms/potential adverse effects
Digestive enzyme inhibitor (Trypsin)	Gas, bloating, pain, diarrhoea
Phytates, bind minerals in gut (e.g. calcium)	Osteoporosis
Goitrogen, supresses thyroid function	Hypothyroidism (under active thyroid)
Isoflavones (phytoestrogens – mimics the female hormone oestrogen)	Hormonal disruption, menstrual cycle disorders, lowers testosterone, endometrial hyperplasia, congenital defects (hypospadias and undescended testes in boys), precocious puberty and breast development in young girls, accelerated brain aging, diminished cognitive ability etc.

Figure 5. Concerns about using soy as a food source.

Source: Keith L., *The Vegetarian Myth*, 2009, p211–229

She goes on to describe the heavily industrialised processes needed to make soy products palatable for human consumption, e.g. soy protein concentrate is manufactured by 'precipitating the solids with aqueous acid, aqueous alcohol, moist heat and/or organic solvents'. The concern is that these extreme industrial processes destroy the very structure of the soy protein, and colours, flavourings and sweeteners are then added to make it palatable.

What about our Second Macronutrient, Protein?

Protein is an organic compound that contains carbon, hydrogen, oxygen and nitrogen. The building blocks of protein are called amino acids and there are 20 different amino acids with each type of protein having a unique combination of amino acids. Nine of the amino acids are essential, meaning that our bodies cannot manufacture them and, therefore, we need to source them from our diet.

All cells and tissues contain protein. Proteins form the structural frames for our muscles, bones, organs, skin and hair. Inside every cell of the body, proteins form part of various functional elements, such as hormones, our immune system's antibodies and enzymes, all of which are involved in a wide range of metabolic interactions. It also provides a storage or carrier function within the body, e.g. the protein haemoglobin carries oxygen to all our cells. Protein is essential for the growth and repair of cells and the maintenance of good health. Since the body does not store excess protein, daily intake is essential to keep us strong and healthy.

Animal products such as meat, poultry, eggs, dairy, and fish are complete sources of protein because they contain all nine essential amino acids. Most plant sources lack essential amino acids. However, soy is a popular plant-based source of protein since it contains all the essential amino acids. Overall, plant proteins are less digestible than animal proteins, more prone to cause allergies and sensitivities (e.g. gluten in wheat and various anti-nutrients in soy – see the previous section) and contain less protein per ounce than animal foods.

And now for the third macronutrient.

Meet the Carbohydrate Family

The simplest form of a carbohydrate is called a 'monosaccharide' or simple sugar, and the most common example is *glucose*, naturally found in fruit and grains. The other two are *fructose* (naturally found in fruit) and *galactose* (found in milk). When two simple sugar molecules combine, we call it a 'disaccharide', for example, glucose + fructose = *sucrose* or *sugar*. When many simple sugars combine, we call it a 'polysaccharide', for example, *starch* = many glucose molecules linked in a chain-like fashion. Examples of starch are grains, pulses, potatoes, and other root vegetables, rice, pasta, and bread.

When we eat, the enzymes in our digestive system break down all food products into their smallest components, so for most carbohydrates, this molecule is glucose. In practical terms, it means that bread, pasta, potatoes, etc. all ultimately break down to glucose, the molecule from which our cells produce energy.

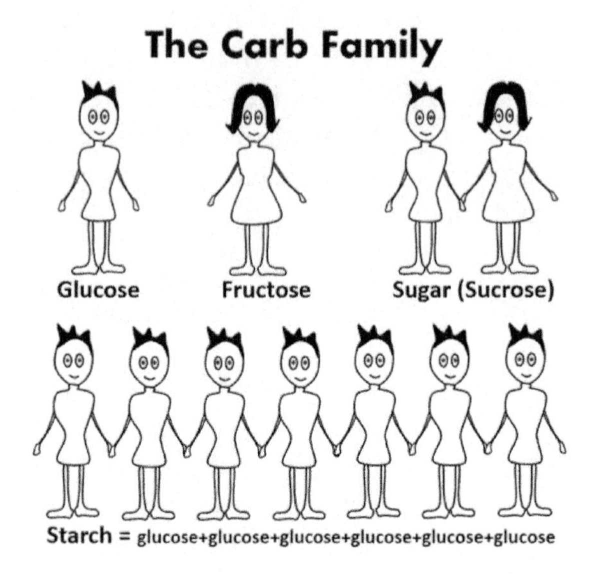

Figure 6. The carb family.

Put another way, if you wish to lose weight by cutting back on your sugar consumption (e.g. not adding sugar to your coffee or tea), but you love eating bread or pasta or cake, you are just kidding yourself! Bread, pasta and cake are all broken down to glucose, which is the same molecule that we find in sugar. Your body doesn't know the difference, because the end products are all the same, i.e. glucose. Believe me, this fact was a game-changer in our self-education process!

What about fructose? Sugar (sucrose) is broken down to one glucose molecule and one fructose molecule. The body handles glucose and fructose slightly differently. After digestion, glucose molecules are taken directly via our bloodstream to our cells where they are used to generate energy for all the cellular processes including the repair and/or building of new cells. Any excess glucose not used in this way is stored by the liver as glycogen or as fat in the liver or abdominal area. Fructose on the other hand doesn't go directly to the cells but is taken up by the liver where it is changed into glucose or storage products (glycogen and/or fat).

So, we can see that both *extra glucose* and *fructose* end up the same way – stored as glycogen or fat!

Getting back to glucose – these molecules *need help* to enter cells for energy production. This helper molecule that guides them from the bloodstream into cells is called *insulin*.

What is Insulin?

When we eat food and our blood sugar level rises, cells in our pancreas are signalled to release the hormone insulin into our bloodstream. Insulin's function is to help glucose molecules enter our cells for energy production. In addition, insulin also helps store excess energy from glucose as glycogen in our liver or muscles or as fat in our liver and abdomen, hence the expression *fat-storage hormone*.

It is, therefore, logical that ongoing high levels of insulin cause weight gain and obesity. Glucose is the molecule that drives the *highest amount of insulin* release in our body. So, the more glucose, the more insulin, the more fat-storage resulting in an expanding waistline and weight gain. Weight management is not a simple question of counting calories, but rather how to balance or in this case *reduce* the level of insulin in our body. It is a hormonal process, that depends on *what* we eat.

↑glucose →↑insulin → ↑fat storage →↑expanding waistline → ↑weight gain

The defect in patients with type 1 diabetes is that their pancreas cannot produce insulin. They need insulin injections to survive. This is very different from people with type 2 diabetes, who can produce insulin; in fact, their insulin levels are usually very high, but their cells are resistant to the effects of insulin (see insulin resistance, in Chapter 4). Because their insulin levels are high, patients with type 2 diabetes carry excess weight or are obese. They do not always require insulin and are often first treated with oral medications. Later in the book, we will propose a different way by which people with type 2 diabetes can address their disease that will lower their requirement to take medication or even completely reverse the condition.

Important Points:

- The constituents of food are divided into macronutrients (*fat, protein and carbohydrates*) and micronutrients (*minerals and vitamins*).
- Of the three macronutrients, only two are *essential*: fat and protein.
- After digestion in our gut, the basic metabolic component of all carbohydrates (sugar and starch) is glucose.
- Fats are either natural – found in unprocessed animal and plant food – or unnatural, i.e. man-made through industrialised processes.
- These industrial processes produce vegetable and seed oils, rich in omega-6, the consumption of which is associated with inflammation in the body and diseases. Global consumption of these products has increased exponentially since the 20th century.
- Animal products such as meat, poultry, eggs, dairy and fish are complete sources of protein because they contain all the essential protein components our body needs.
- Unfermented soy products contain various anti-nutrients (e.g. isoflavones and goitrogens) associated with a range of conditions including developmental abnormalities and underactive thyroid disease.

Chapter 2

WHAT DID OUR ANCESTORS EAT?

'The only source of knowledge is experience.'

Albert Einstein

In the Western world, we have all been indoctrinated with the idea that a balanced diet is the best way to stay healthy. As mentioned earlier this very often means a diet comprising fruits and vegetables, including nuts and grains, with only limited amounts of meat (in fact the less meat and fat you eat the better). A plate filled with a variety of colourful food, five-a-day, etc. comes to mind. This is contrary to what happened in the past.

At school, we learned that in previous centuries sailors, miners and explorers frequently died of scurvy because of a lack of fresh vegetables and fruits. Scurvy is a disease that develops as a result of a lack of vitamin C (or ascorbic acid).

Examples from Nature

Is this how things work in nature? Do animals generally eat a great variety of food types? We all agree that animals living in the wild are in good health when they live in their natural habitat. But they don't all eat the same food, even if they share a habitat. In Africa, giraffe and lions share the same habitat, but their diets are completely different. And so is the diet of the koala living in Australia. All three species eat the following exclusively: giraffes eat acacia leaves, lions eat meat, and koalas feast on eucalyptus leaves.

The food animals eat is determined by the anatomical differences in their gut and, if they cannot find the correct food, they will become sick and eventually die. Each species can, therefore, eat only foods for which it is genetically and anatomically programmed. Just like humans.

So, what about humans then? Did they always happily feast on fruits and vegetables whilst enjoying a life free from chronic diseases, unlike today?

What did our Ancestors Eat?

Humans developed as hunter-gatherers and obtained their food by hunting, fishing, scavenging and gathering wild plants and other edibles. These prehistoric societies relied on the bounty of nature and often lived in groups of a few dozen people, consisting of several family units. In northern Europe particularly, the hunter-gatherers lived largely on mammoths because they had so much fat in them. These animals were hunted to extinction by humans.

About 10,000 to 15,000 years ago humans began to domesticate animals and to cultivate grasses (the precursors of our modern cereals, including wheat and barley). Domesticated grains were a new addition to the human diet, reducing our ancestors' reliance on hunting, fishing and gathering. The focus on agriculture changed the diet composition from a predominantly meat-based diet (75 per cent) to a high-carbohydrate agricultural diet.

It, therefore, came as a big surprise just over a hundred years ago, when the Arctic explorer Vilhjalmur Stefansson, who lived with the Inuit (Eskimos) in the Mackenzie River area of the Canadian Arctic in 1906, reported that he (as did his hosts) exclusively lived on fish and meat for a whole year without suffering any illness like scurvy. It is estimated that 70 to 80 per cent of their diet came from animal fat.

An account of his experience *'Adventures in Diet'* was published by Harper's Monthly Magazine in 1935. Being an Arctic explorer, he knew and met men who participated in other historical expeditions. For instance, his article provides fascinating insights into Robert Scott's second Antarctic expedition. Scott and four companions failed to return after reaching the South Pole in 1912. Scurvy weakened Scott and his men 'on their return journey and progressed so rapidly that the growing weakness prevented them, if only by ten miles, from being able to get back to the final provision depot'. Scott had received standard medical advice on the prevention of scurvy before he left Britain, which was to rely on lime juice, fruits and marmalade.

This was in contrast to Ernest Shackleton's Antarctic expedition a few years later when his ship became entrapped in pack ice. He and his men all survived the ordeal without 'a sign of scurvy; every man retained his full strength' as reported by Dr Alister Forbes Mackay, a physician from Edinburgh, who was a member of the expedition and later the physician on one of Stefansson's own expeditions. Dr Mackay attributed the survival of Shackleton and his men mainly to the fact that half the food they consumed during their stay in the Antarctic was fresh meat from penguins and seals.

Although Stefansson acknowledges that the amount of vitamin C in fruit and vegetables is high, vitamin C levels deteriorate rapidly over time and, in the long Arctic journeys, would not have sustained the levels needed to prevent scurvy. His view was that since the human body only needs a tiny amount of vitamin C that a diet of some fresh meat daily (not overcooked) is alone sufficient to prevent scurvy. Certainly, his own experience in the Arctic, as well as that of Shackleton and his men, provide historic evidence for this.

It is not only the Eskimos or Ernest Shackleton and his men who were able to survive solely on an animal-based diet. Teicholz, in her book

The Big Fat Surprise, describes several other examples, e.g. George Mann, a doctor and professor of biochemistry from Vanderbilt University, who took a mobile laboratory to Kenya in the 1960s to study the Masai people. Their daily diet comprised *meat and a few litres of milk* (sometimes mixed with cow's blood). The Masai considered fruits and vegetables fit only to be eaten by cows! This meant that animal fat (mostly saturated fat) was the source of more than 60 per cent of their daily calorie intake. Despite this, Mann found that the Masai are slender of build, their blood pressure was relatively low by Western standards, their blood cholesterol values were low, while no chronic diseases such as cancer and diabetes were found after performing 50 autopsies.

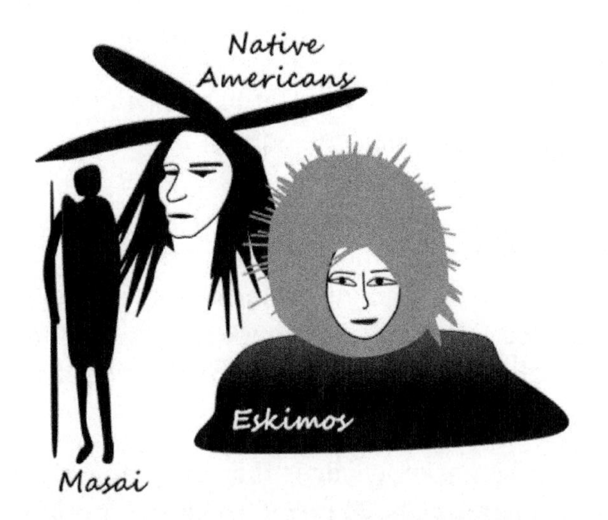

Another example is the Native American tribes who were extraordinarily successful hunters, adept at trapping and killing with bow and arrow. They ate fish, clams and buffalo meat. The late-nineteenth, early-twentieth-century physician and anthropologist Aleš Hrdlička, after examining more than two thousand Native Americans, found them clinically to have been spectacularly healthy and to have lived to a ripe old age.

Unfortunately, this picture of health and prosperity changed as Europeans settled in the Indian territories. Several factors impacted the traditional Native American's way of life. When the Europeans came, they hunted game to near extinction and their farming methods impacted the local environment to such an extent that it drove tribes to famine, starvation and despair. The trading posts they established supplied tribes with sugar, coffee and canned goods which soon replaced their traditional foodstuffs. In his book *Why We Get Fat*, Gary Taubes mentions that the Pima Native American tribe from Arizona may have the highest incidence of obesity and diabetes in the United States today.

The same pattern of events was repeated in other geographical areas; e.g. the European colonists of Africa, India and Australia found little clinical evidence of chronic degenerative diseases including cancer in the local populations they encountered. The sad truth is that, when these indigenous societies began adopting a Western diet (high levels of carbohydrates) in the twentieth century, they started to develop all the chronic degenerative diseases so prevalent today.

If our modern concept is correct that meat and fat are bad for us, then how do we explain the exceptional health these traditional societies experienced for millennia? Clearly, we need to question our nutritional beliefs and face up to the fact that what we think is healthy and what really is healthy may not be the same.

Ancient/Traditional versus Modern Day Diet Composition

Let's reflect on this for a moment. The main difference between our ancestor's diet and our modern diet is the proportional contribution of the three macronutrients. Figure 7 gives a comparison between a pre-agricultural diet vs our modern Western diet. We can see that protein consumption remains fairly constant, making fat and carbohydrates the two variants.

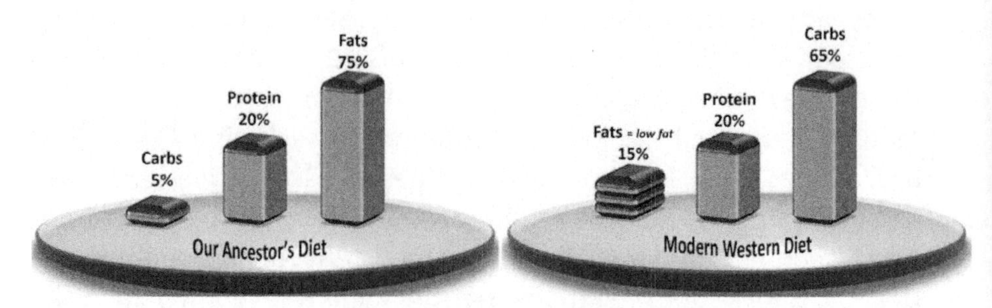

Figure 7. Composition of Ancient/Traditional vs Modern diet (based on the UK Eatwell Guide).

Our modern diet contains a high concentration of carbohydrates, which is the exact opposite of what our ancestors consumed. Traditionally, fat was the most important and abundant macronutrient in the diet. In modern-day society, it is the reverse, with fat making the smallest contribution to our diet. Furthermore, the fat we eat is unnatural because it is a 'low-fat' version – not something that we find in nature because it is modified by industry, i.e. man-made.

This highlights another point: our ancestors ate an animal-based diet providing all the fat and protein they needed. At the beginning of the first chapter, we saw that fat and protein are the only essential macronutrients, hence throughout human evolution, our hominid ancestors and later traditional *Homo sapiens* societies developed and followed a diet that not only sustained them but also allowed them to lead a healthy life without the burden of chronic degenerative diseases.

This way of living was 'lost' after four to six million years in the twentieth century, when scientists started blaming fat, the most important macronutrient that sustained human life, as the cause of chronic illness, particularly heart disease. Since then our diet has progressively changed to a predominantly plant-based one, which is driving the high levels of carbohydrate consumption – ironically the only macronutrient which is nonessential.

Animal products = fat + protein
Plant products = carbohydrates + protein

We need to understand why the subject of nutrition has become so controversial. Why for thousands of years humankind knew instinctively what to eat and why in today's world we are confused by several conflicting views from news flashes and advertisements advising us daily on what the best new products are to eat. Is it a surprise then that most people don't know what to believe or who to trust? The next chapter will delve into the reasons why nutrition has become such a controversial subject.

Important Points:

- Our pre-agricultural ancestors ate an animal-based diet providing all the nutrients they needed and did not suffer from lifestyle diseases.
- Modern-day humans eat a diet predominantly consisting of carbohydrates, which includes an array of highly processed foods and drinks.
- Numerous traditional societies adopted a Western diet in the twentieth century and subsequently developed chronic degenerative diseases.

Chapter 3

THE WAR BETWEEN FAT AND SUGAR

and how it impacts the lives of millions around the globe

'Seldom in medical history has there been a more catastrophic result of such scientific dishonesty.'

Professor Tim Noakes

Fat, Cholesterol and Sugar: Where did it all Start?

The fat/sugar controversy involved many scientists over at least seven decades and following their arguments, deceptions, fabrications and misrepresentations makes for fascinating reading. For the sake of brevity and clarity, we will concentrate on the two main players in this debate. Nevertheless, for those who would like to review a more comprehensive and detailed history of events, refer to the Reference section at the end of the book.

Our two main protagonists are 'Anti-Fat' represented by Ancel Keys and 'Anti-Sugar' represented by John Yudkin.

John Yudkin identified added sugars as the primary agent of lifestyle diseases, whilst Ancel Keys identified total fat, saturated fat and dietary cholesterol as the culprits. However, by the 1980s, few scientists believed that added sugars played a significant role in heart disease, and the first 1980 *Dietary Guidelines for Americans* focused on reducing total fat, saturated fat and dietary cholesterol for heart disease prevention.

But we are getting ahead of ourselves.

Fat, or Rather, Saturated Fat

Ancel Keys, an American physiologist received his first PhD in 1930 in oceanography and biology from the University of California, Berkeley, and his second PhD, in physiology, from Cambridge in 1936. Particularly of interest is the fact that he had no training in medicine or cardiology or epidemiology.

In 1948, the American Heart Association began a multimillion-dollar campaign to raise money for heart-disease research, because so many Americans were dying of heart attacks (Gary Taubes, *The Case Against Sugar*). This provided a unique opportunity for scientists to follow the money into heart disease research.

A few years later, in 1953, Keys, then at the University of Minnesota, proposed that too much cholesterol and fat in the diet was the key driver of heart disease. In support of his statement, he included data from six countries showing a direct relationship between the amount of fat in the diet and the number of deaths from heart disease.

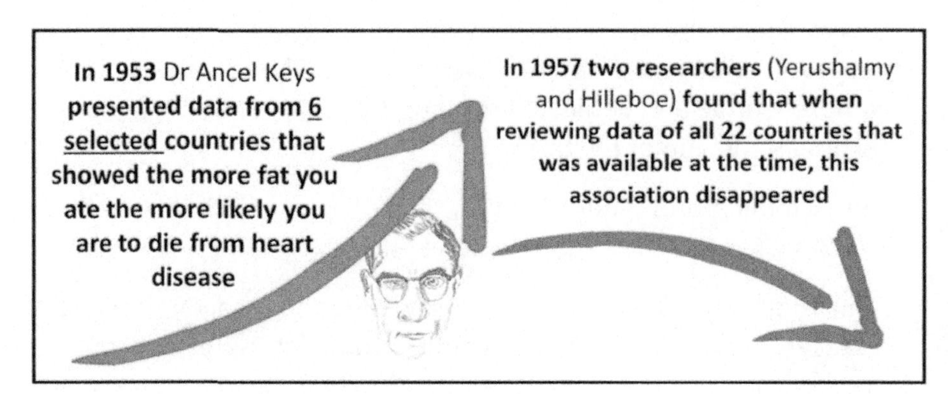

Keys was heavily criticized by two researchers, Yerushalmy and Hilleboe, for cherry-picking six countries from the 22 on which data was available at the time. We don't know why Keys only selected six countries but, since the positive association between fat and heart disease disappears when data from the 22 countries are included, one can but speculate that there was devious intent. Such a targeted selection of data to show association, of course, amounts to scientific cheating.

This criticism did not deter Keys, and, maybe because of it, he then embarked on his 'Seven Countries Study (SCS)' for which, again, as for his six countries study, he did not employ random selection. The study by all accounts was flawed, sloppy and conducted without the necessary scientific rigour.

In her book, *The Big Fat Surprise,* Nina Teicholz provides a detailed account of issues relating to the study. To name a few – the study took no notice of differences in the physical activity of participants, there was no consistency in how dietary data were collected from the different nations participating (for example, in the US, one day's data was collected from 1.5 per cent of men, while in other countries, data was collected for a period up to seven days), less than 4 per cent (499 of 12,770 participants) of dietary data from *all participants* was analysed, 60 per cent of the Greek participants from Crete were fasting during the survey and different chemical methods were used to analyse the fat content in food samples. Smoking, one of the key factors associated with heart disease, was not considered at all!

One wonders how a serious scientist could truthfully come to any conclusions based on the degree of variability associated with almost every aspect of the study and then compound that by finally analysing only a fraction of the data collected. Teicholz mentions in her book that, years later, in 1999, the Seven Countries study's lead Italian researcher Alessandro Menotti revisited the data. He found that the food that correlated most closely with deaths from heart disease was not saturated fat but sugar.

In January 1961, Keys made the cover of Time Magazine and, in the article, explained how elevated blood cholesterol concentrations directly cause coronary atherosclerosis: 'Americans eat too much fat. With meat, milk, butter and ice cream, the calorie-heavy U.S. diet is 40 per cent fat, and most of that is saturated fat—the insidious kind, that increases blood cholesterol, damages arteries, and leads to coronary disease.'

If this wasn't enough to instil *lipophilia*, (the fear of fat), nothing would.

Onwards and upwards – Keys was definitely not for stopping.

An even bigger study followed, of which Keys was a principal investigator, conducted from 1968 to 1973: the Minnesota Coronary Experiment (MCE). The topic of investigation was whether a cholesterol-lowering diet, which replaced saturated fat in the diet with vegetable oil (corn oil, an omega-6 polyunsaturated fat), would decrease heart disease and death related to cardiovascular disease. The study included 9,570 men and women.

Although the original findings of the study were available in 1976, the final results were reported only thirteen years later, in 1989. It stated that there were no differences between the saturated fat and vegetable oil groups for heart disease, death from heart disease or overall death rate.

In 2016, twenty-seven years after the initial publication of the results and 12 years after Keys' death, a reanalysis of the data was published in *The British Medical Journal* (Ramsden et al., *The BMJ*) which revealed that the results published were incomplete and incorrect. That was a full 40 years after the original results became available. The reanalysis showed that the survival of participants over 65 years old receiving corn oil was significantly worse compared to the control group of participants who continued to eat their usual saturated fat diet. *Thus, the results did not support the original hypothesis that saturated fat causes heart disease. Instead, it showed that saturated fat had absolutely no effect on heart disease outcomes.*

One can but speculate what would have happened if the true results of the MCE study had been revealed in 1976. Might it have prevented the harmful dietary advice and guidelines that were subsequently developed, in particular the 1977 U.S. Dietary Guidelines developed by Senator George McGovern's hopelessly under-qualified committee (see later)?

Yet, the facts were not known at the time, and, throughout the 1960s, Keys became more and more influential by securing places for himself and his allies on the boards of the most powerful bodies in American healthcare, including the American Heart Association and the National Institutes of Health. These powerful allies tipped the tables in his favour.

Here was a man with an unwavering belief in his own hypothesis and, even in the face of conflicting evidence, willing to bury or ignore inconvenient results that strayed from sound and responsible scientific principles.

Where Does this Leave us with Cholesterol?

Let's go back to Keys' Time Magazine interview in 1961. He reported, 'As the fatty protein molecules travel in the bloodstream, they are deposited in the intima, or inner wall, of a coronary artery. The proteins and fats are burned off, and the cholesterol is left behind. As cholesterol piles up, it narrows, irritates and damages the artery, encouraging the formation of calcium deposits and slowing circulation. Eventually, one of two things happens. A clot forms at the site, seals off the flow of blood to the heart and provokes a heart attack. Or the deposits themselves get so big that they choke off the artery's flow to the point that an infarct occurs: the heart muscle is suffocated, cells supplied by the artery die, and the heart is permanently, perhaps fatally, injured'.

The importance of the Time Magazine article cannot be underestimated. It presented Keys' hypothesis to the world as if it was proven and fact.

So, what is cholesterol, you may ask? Is it also a fat?

The answer is NO.

Cholesterol and fats are not the same. They are not even 'related' biochemically. That means their biochemical structure is completely different and the one doesn't morph into the other.

Cholesterol is not a saturated fat

The only connection is that foods (usually from animal sources) containing cholesterol also tend to contain fats, specifically saturated fat, a basic nutritional fact that Dr Malcolm Kendrick points out in his book, *The Great Cholesterol Con*.

What is true about cholesterol is that it is a *vital substance* for the body. Without cholesterol in our bodies, we cannot live (see Figure 8). Our bodies absorb cholesterol from the food we eat but also make cholesterol in our liver and brain to ensure that all the critical processes in the body are being supported.

The obvious question to ask is: If it is so important, even essential for our survival, why would it lead to heart disease and death? And further, why did Keys make it part of his heart disease hypothesis? The question is still being debated by scholars today.

We have already mentioned that both the Six and Seven Countries Studies as well as the MCE study that Keys undertook all failed to prove that fat/cholesterol promotes heart disease. In fact, it showed the reverse.

Functions of Cholesterol in the Body

Cholesterol is vital because

- it is necessary for hormone production.
- it makes bile acids to help with digestion.
- it is part of the membrane of every single cell in our body.
- our brain needs 25% of all the cholesterol in our body to function normally (e.g. memory, learning etc.).
- it is critical for our bones - needed to make vitamin D in our skin.

Figure 8. Functions of cholesterol in the body.

On several occasions throughout his life, Keys himself confirmed that dietary intake was unrelated to blood cholesterol concentration. In 1991, he wrote in the *New England Journal of Medicine (NEJM)* that a man who ate 25 eggs a day had a normal cholesterol level. Prof Tim Noakes mentions in *CrossFit: It's the Insulin Resistance, Stupid: Part 9* that Keys made the following comment seven years before his death in 2004: 'There's no connection whatsoever between cholesterol in food and cholesterol in blood. And we've known that all along. Cholesterol in the diet doesn't matter at all unless you happen to be a chicken or a rabbit.'

In 2010, British obesity and nutrition researcher Dr Zoë Harcombe performed an analysis of the World Health Organisation data on cholesterol levels for 192 countries around the world and found that *lower blood cholesterol* values correlated with *higher rates of death from heart disease as well as all causes of death.* She then performed a review (meta-analysis) of all randomly controlled studies from the 1960s up to 2016, the aim of which was to lower heart disease by limiting the intake of dietary fat. She concluded that there was no data to support this theory. The studies included in the analysis involved nearly 90,000 participants in total with a mean follow-up period of almost 12 years.

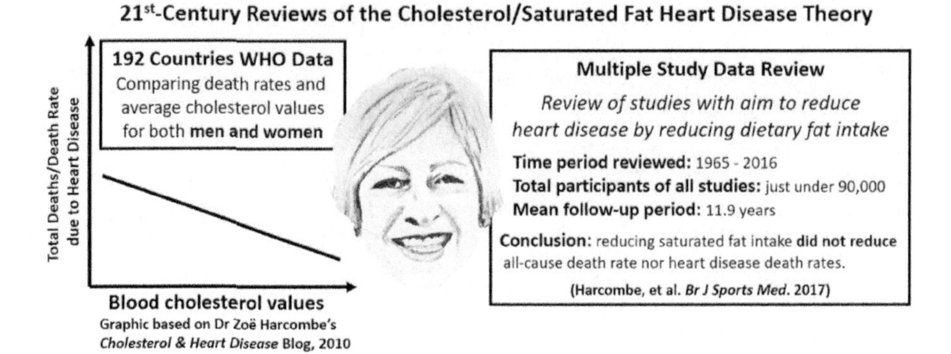

Figure 9. 21st-century reviews of the cholesterol/saturated fat heart disease theory.

In summary, the scientific data is clear: the saturated fat/cholesterol theory is false. Neither saturated fat nor cholesterol is related to heart disease or an increased risk of dying early. So why is it then still today regarded as the absolute truth, with millions of people worldwide believing that they need to lower their cholesterol by taking statins and to reduce their intake of food rich in cholesterol, such as eggs and seafood?

Because their doctors, the media and all the respectable health bodies tell them to do so.

The pharmaceutical industry took its cue from Keys in the 1950s that cholesterol was an undesirable substance that had to be kept at bay. That provided them with a 'target molecule' and all they had to do was to find something that would block the manufacturing process of cholesterol in our liver and our brain. They started working on cholesterol-lowering drugs or statins as they became known in the 1950s. The first statin, discovered in the 1970s, was called lovastatin and was released on the market in 1987 (Mevacor, from Merck). Many more statins have been released by various pharmaceutical companies since then.

Global statin usage has exploded since its initial release and is driven forward by the National Cholesterol Education Program (NCEP) guidance through progressively ratcheting 'ideal' cholesterol blood levels lower and lower and simultaneously increasing the number of people now eligible to be offered the 'treatment'. Total global sales are on track to reach an estimated $1 trillion in 2020.

As far as I am aware, this is the first time in medical history that a vital natural chemical molecule has been so vilified. The pharmaceutical industry has the licence to develop these weapons of mass destruction (statins) that lower the level of this 'undesirable' vital substance in our bodies and have an army of soldiers ready to deploy it (medical practitioners across the world).

While statins are a mega business, the pharmaceutical industry is not keen to dwell on the serious side-effects associated with these drugs. Once again, anything that can impact business is kept quiet and very seldom referred to. I often ask people on statin treatment if, prior to prescription, their GP mentioned the potential side effects of the treatment? To date, not a single person has replied in the affirmative. To name but a few of the side effects: can cause type 2 diabetes; can increase your blood pressure and cause heart failure, memory loss and disorientation; can cause muscle pains and weakness, joint pains, cataract development, neuropathy and cancer; and is contraindicated in pregnancy due to severe birth defects (limb, heart and nervous system abnormalities).

After all of this, the troubling question is why is our medical profession so keen to prescribe this treatment? There are many potential answers to this question. To name a few: misinformation, ignorance and misrepresentation of clinical trial results. Let me give you an example of how the industry can easily manipulate data from clinical trials to portray the results in a very favourable light.

Clinical trials usually involve the comparison of the effect of a drug versus no-drug in two randomly selected groups of people. The outcomes of the study then quantify how much better or worse the treatment group is when compared to the control group. These results are then expressed as an absolute or relative risk (usually as a per cent value). To demonstrate this point, Figure 10 gives a simplified version of how clinical trial results can be presented to create a completely different impression from the real value or benefit.

Clinical Trials: Relative versus Absolute Risk Example

	Treatment Group 1 + Drug	Control Group 1 No Drug	Treatment Group 2 + Drug	Control Group 2 No Drug
Number participants	100	100	1000	1000
Number of deaths	1	2	1	2
Percentage	1%	2%	0.1%	0.2%
Relative Risk		50% increase		50% increase
Absolute Risk		Additional 1/100 patients not receiving treatment will die		Additional 1/1000 patients not receiving treatment will die

Figure 10. Clinical trials: Relative vs absolute risk example.

For example, in *A Statin Nation*, Dr Malcolm Kendrick provides the following example: the statin Lipitor was marketed by Pfizer in the US claiming that it reduces the risk of heart attack by 36 per cent. That was the relative risk analysis. When determining the absolute number of heart attacks, it was 1.1 per cent, meaning that 98.9 per cent of those taking the drug for 5 years did not benefit (0.2 per cent reduction per year of treatment). Most medical doctors are oblivious of the cunning way in which the pharmaceutical companies present their promotional material and unquestioningly assume that the data shown is, in fact, the absolute risk.

Author and UK cardiologist, Dr Aseem Malhotra, writes in *The Pioppi Diet*, 'If you haven't had a heart attack, and you don't suffer from heart disease, taking a cholesterol-lowering statin pill will not prolong your life by one day.'

Sugar

As mentioned at the beginning of the chapter, from the late 1950s to the early 1970s, Ancel Keys and John Yudkin, a British physiologist and nutritionist, had an ongoing debate in the scientific literature regarding the idea that sugar is an alternative dietary explanation as a cause of heart disease.

John Yudkin was born in London in 1910 to immigrant Russian Jewish parents. His father died when he was young and his mother brought up her five sons in poverty. After school, a scholarship enabled him to study biochemistry and physiology, and later medicine, at Cambridge. During the Second World War, he served in the Royal Army Medical Corps, and post-war became a professor at Queen Elizabeth College in London, where he built a department of nutrition science with an international reputation.

He focused his research on the effects of sugar using a series of laboratory experiments on animals and humans and observed, as others had before him, that sugar is processed in the liver where it turns to fat before entering the bloodstream.

In 1957, Yudkin suggested that Keys had perhaps overlooked any possible effects of high sugar intake in persons living in countries in which dietary fat intake was also high. He was aware of the dramatic rise over the last two hundred years in the amount of sugar consumed in the UK and the US, and commented, 'We now eat in two weeks the amount of sugar our ancestors of 200 years ago ate in a whole year.' That was a 25-fold increase in consumption!

The development of sugar plantations in the Caribbean, made possible by the slave trade, was the main driving force for the ever-increasing sugar consumption. Two dips in consumption occurred in the 20th century with the two world wars (due to sugar rationing), but the escalating trend soon corrected itself at the end of each war with a staggering estimated consumption of 70 kg (155 pounds) per person per year by the turn of the century in 2000.

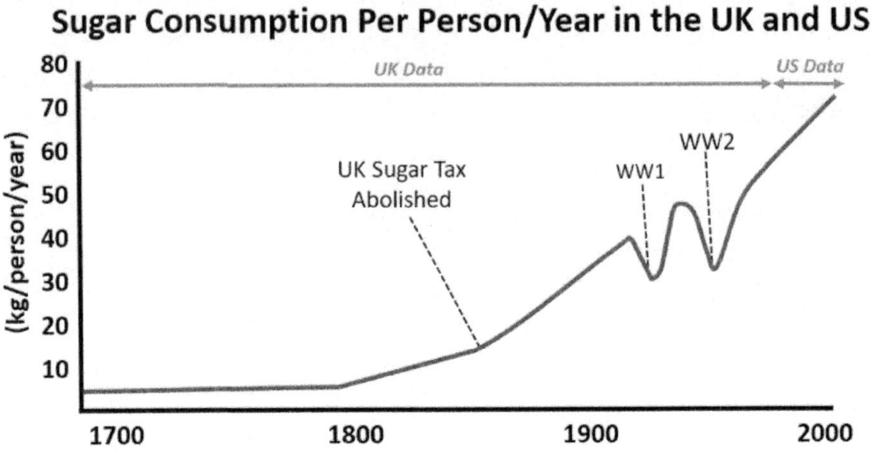

Figure 11. Sugar consumption per person/year in the UK and the US.

Based on: Yudkin J., *Pure, White and Deadly* and Johnson R.J. et al., Potential role of sugar (fructose) in the epidemic of hypertension, obesity and the metabolic syndrome, diabetes, kidney disease, and cardiovascular disease. *Am J Clin Nutr*, 2007; 86:901.

Based on observations from different countries across the globe, Yudkin and his supporters suspected that sugar was the prime suspect in the rising epidemics of obesity, diabetes, hypertension and heart disease. His view was bolstered by reports from Israel, South Africa and the South Pacific linking sugar intake to epidemic increases in numbers for diabetes.

T. L. Cleave, in *The Saccharine Disease*, reports observations from Dr George Campbell, a South African physician, about the very high incidence of diabetes in immigrants from India working in sugar plantations in KwaZulu-Natal. Their consumption of sugar was nearly 80 pounds per year, while in India where the prevalence for diabetes was much lower (one in a hundred), sugar consumption was estimated at only 12 pounds per year.

Campbell himself published data in 1963, showing a similar difference in diabetes prevalence between the urban and rural Zulu populations of KwaZulu-Natal, where the city dwellers had a much higher sugar consumption. From their medical histories, he observed a remarkably constant interval of 20 years for these migrants to the cities to develop diabetes and 30 years for heart disease to manifest itself. Tooth decay, periodontal disease, and gout, often preceded the development of diabetes and hypertension.

Nevertheless, Keys did not take kindly to Yudkin's criticism and attacked and ridiculed his sugar theory as 'a mountain of nonsense'. He accused him of propaganda. 'Yudkin and his commercial backers are not deterred by the facts,' he said. 'They continue to sing the same discredited tune.'

Keys' personal attack was ironic, taking into account that he himself was funded by the sugar industry. Therefore, it was Keys and his commercial backers who had a vested interest in minimising any links between sugar and chronic diseases. Yudkin was a mild-mannered man, always polite, and did not respond in kind. He ultimately paid a high price for his own personal aversion or inability to enter the field of scientific political combat, especially when facing a powerful, politically savvy animal like Keys. As seen earlier in the chapter, Keys became a very powerful opponent throughout the 1960s through his associations with major American funding agencies.

Yudkin was progressively marginalised and discredited by prominent nutritionists supporting Keys as well as the food industry, which relied heavily on sugar additives in the preparation of processed food and drinks. He found himself disinvited from international nutrition conferences, while research journals refused to publish his papers.

Yudkin retired from his academic position in 1971, and in 1972, his book on the dangers of sugar, *Pure, White and Deadly*, was published. In the book, he complains about the money that the sugar industry spent on advertising and public relations, whilst they, at the same time, denied that sugar was harmful to heart health and health in general. He died in 1995, a disappointed, largely forgotten man.

In 2015 and 2016, the New York Times published two articles (*Coca-Cola Funds Effort to Alter Obesity Battle* and *Sugar Backers Paid to Shift Blame to Fat*) reporting how the food, drink and sugar industries paid researchers to confuse the public and deflect attention from processed food and beverage intake to a lack of exercise as the main culprit driving obesity (in other words, shifting blame from their products to an inherent 'weakness' afflicting the consumer public). The unhealthy relationship between the American Society for Nutrition and the Academy of Nutrition and Dietetics with companies such as Kraft Foods, McDonald's, PepsiCo and Hershey's was also revealed.

Manipulation of Research through Funding by the Sugar, Food and Drink Industries

2015 and 2016 New York Times articles revealed Coca-Cola & Sugar Association provided millions $$$ funding to US-based researchers to

- minimise the link between sugar and obesity/heart health and
- instead shift blame on to the role of saturated fat and lack of exercise.

In 1965, three Harvard scientists published a paper in the *New England Journal of Medicine (NEJM)*, advancing the theory that fat (not sugar) is responsible for heart disease. In 2016, it came to light that the Sugar Association paid them about $50,000 in today's $ to publish the review *(NEJM.1965;277:245-7, JAMA Intern Med. 2016;176:1680-1685).*

Figure 12. Manipulation of research by the sugar, food and drink industries.

It is clear that, from the 1970s, the anti-sugar activists had lost the battle. The fat/cholesterol activists and food industry have shaped the opinions of the public health authorities and governments of the West on the healthy features of sugar and the detrimental effects of fat and cholesterol.

That was until 2009 when the American paediatric endocrinologist Robert Lustig became interested in Yudkin's work. Lustig became very concerned about the obesity epidemic he was witnessing in babies and children and the devastating role played by added sugar and high fructose corn syrup in processed foods. It is only after Yudkin's death that his contributions are being valued through support from Lustig as well as the brilliant research of two investigative journalists, Gary Taubes (*Good Calories, Bad Calories, The Case Against Sugar*) and Nina Teicholz (*The Big Fat Surprise*), who were brave enough to take on the dogmatic evidence-averse medical and nutritionist fraternities.

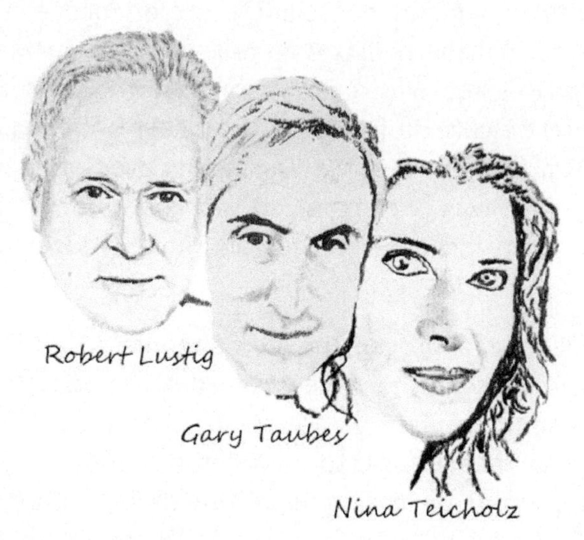

Consequences of the Fat–Sugar War

After the Second World War, nobody could have foreseen the devastating impact that the nutritional disagreement about the cause of heart disease would have on human health.

Government Implements Nutrition Guidelines

In the late 1970s in America, plant-based diets were starting to gain more traction in the popular consciousness with the one contributing factor being the demonisation of saturated fat which had been underway by then for almost 20 years.

At the same time, politicians in America became interested in the question of what people should eat, and, for the first time in history, a government mandated the ideal diet for its citizens. It started in

1977 when the Senate Select Committee on Nutrition and Human Needs led by Senator George McGovern made recommendations for the composition of a healthy diet: reduced fat intake from 40 to 30 per cent (saturated fat capped at 10 per cent) of calories with an increase in carbohydrate to 55 to 60 per cent of calories.

The committee staff had no scientific experience – it comprised lawyers and former journalists who relied heavily on Mark Hegsted for guidance. Hegsted was a professor of nutrition at the Harvard School of Public Health, a friend of Ancel Keys and co-author of the 1965 *New England Journal of Medicine* paper promoting the fat-heart disease theory. It was later revealed that the authors of this paper received a cash incentive from the Sugar Association for its publication.

Although Congress approved the 'components' of a healthy diet, a group of scientists at the time was adamant that the evidence condemning saturated fat was not persuasive. Yet the Senate report stated, 'We cannot afford to await the ultimate proof before correcting trends we believe to be detrimental.' In 1980, the *Dietary Guidelines for Americans* were published and became the basis of the USDA food pyramid, 'My Plate', and were adopted in the UK in 1983 as the 'Eatwell Guide'. Other English-speaking countries around the globe followed suit.

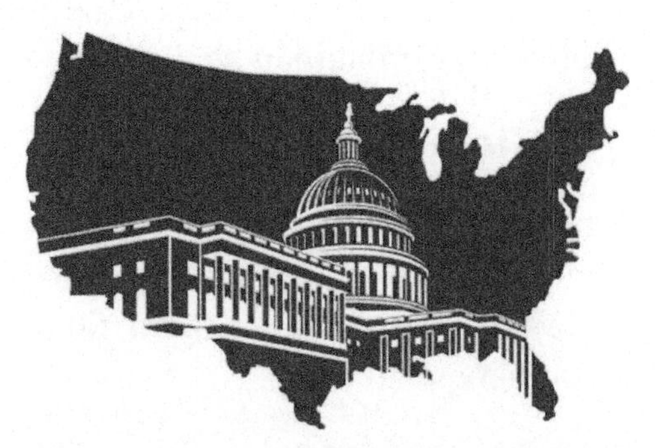

The US Senate Select Committee on Nutrition and Human Needs made recommendations about the composition of a healthy diet, which ultimately resulted in the publication of the *Dietary Guidelines for Americans* in 1980.

Today, 40 years later, we are still awaiting the 'ultimate proof' for the fat/cholesterol-heart theory. Yet, a different kind of proof has become blatantly obvious on a global scale: the massive increase in the prevalence of obesity, diabetes, high blood pressure and dementia. See Figure 13 for the prevalence trends in the US for obesity, high blood pressure (hypertension) and diabetes since 1900. For all three conditions, there has been a steep increase in percentage rates since 1980 when the guidelines were first introduced in the US.

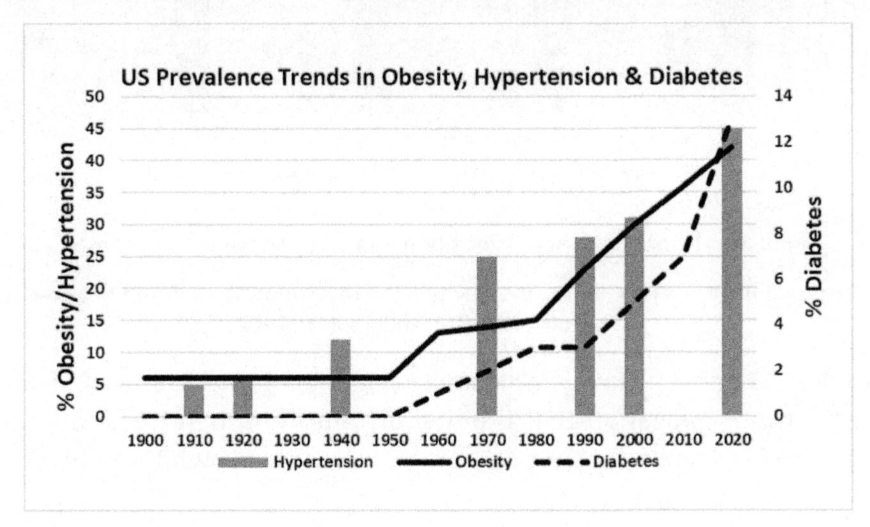

Figure 13. US prevalence trends in obesity, hypertension and diabetes.

Data sources: Gross L. S. et al, 2004; Johnson R. J. et al., 2007; Hales et al., 2020; CDC Diabetes Data and Statistics; National Center for Health Statistics, National Health and Nutrition Examination Survey, 2013–2016.

The obvious question is: How did the macronutrient composition of the American diet change after the Dietary Guidelines were introduced in 1980? The answer can be found in data collected by the CDC from 1971 to 2000. During this period, increased calorie intake was primarily due to carbohydrate intake; there was a slight decrease in protein intake with a definite decrease in fat intake. Spot on! The data confirmed that the American public was paying attention to the new guidelines and was changing their eating habits accordingly.

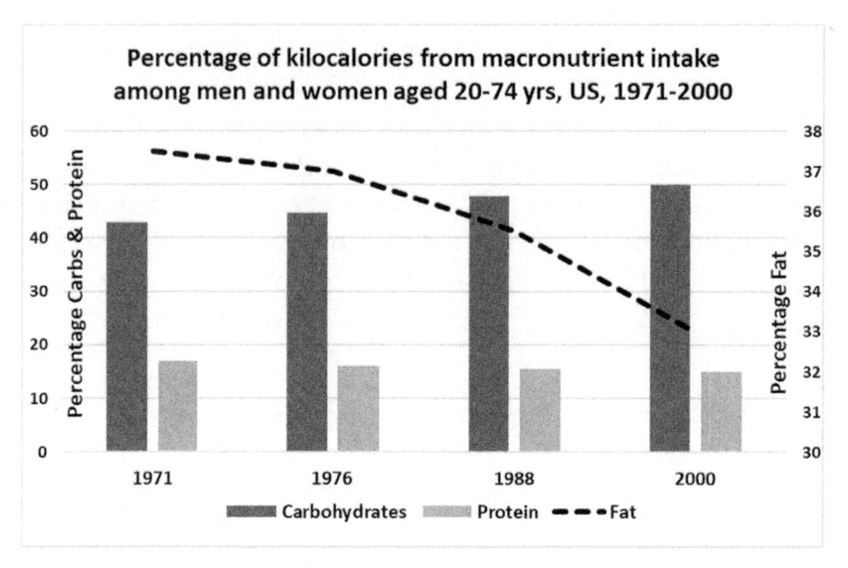

Figure 14. US macronutrient kilocalorie intake among men and women.

Redrawn from: Trends in intake of energy and macronutrients – United States, 1971–2000, *MMWR*. 2004;53(4):80–82.

Figures 13 and 14 provide a clear visual comparison of trends and are yet another indication that obesity, diabetes and heart disease are not related to fat intake, but associated with increased carbohydrate/sugar consumption.

The two dietary components with the greatest increase in consumption in the twentieth century are sugar and shortening. Shortening is the term used for hydrogenated vegetable oil products (see Chapter 1), with soybean oil making the largest contribution to this category. The increase in both commodities in the last half of the twentieth century was dramatic. The production of both products requires heavily industrialised processes and is completely artificial. The end products themselves and all the added chemicals used in the production may have an impact on the health of consumers, which is of great concern.

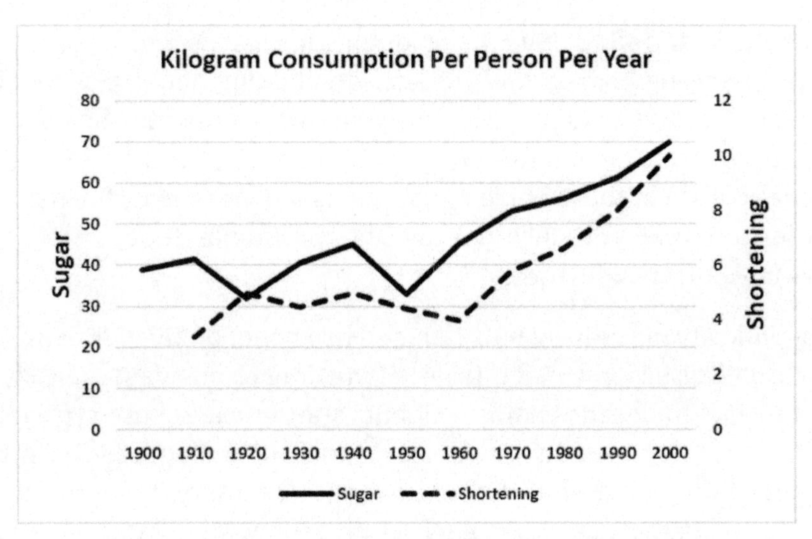

Figure 15. Changes in consumption of sugar and shortening. Redrawn from: Blasbalg et al., *Am J Clin Nutr*, 2011, and Yudkin J., 2016: *Pure, White and Deadly*.

New Epidemics Emerge

From the 1980s onwards, the lives of millions of people, initially starting in the US and then spreading to other Western countries and ultimately most countries in the world, have been affected by an epidemic increase in obesity, diabetes, heart disease, cancer, dementia and many other conditions.

With sugar being exonerated from any blame, the food and drink industry had the freedom to exploit the addictive properties of sugar in an ever-expanding array of new and enticing products, aiming at all age groups including babies and young children. The products were and are creating an ever-increasing global cohort of 'sugarholics', all of whom believe the cunning advertisements claiming that the products are healthy because of their 'low-fat properties'. Sugar makes low-fat food more palatable.

Sugar now started to drive the epidemics in lifestyle diseases that are ever-increasing and, in the process, dominating and overwhelming our health care systems. Governments are increasing their health care budgets, but it is like pouring money into a big black hole because the real cause of these epidemics is not acknowledged by the medical profession and certainly not by the profitable food, drink and pharmaceutical industries.

The difficulty in studying nutrition and its impact on the development of chronic diseases is that it takes a long time to manifest clinically. It takes years to decades before patients start to experience symptoms from these diseases. As we've seen earlier in this chapter from the clinical data collected in the mid-twentieth century in South Africa, type 2 diabetes takes 20 years to present with symptoms, heart disease 30 years, while cancer and dementia can take much longer. Typically, nutrition studies only last a few years which is too short to give a true reflection of the long-term situation or outcomes.

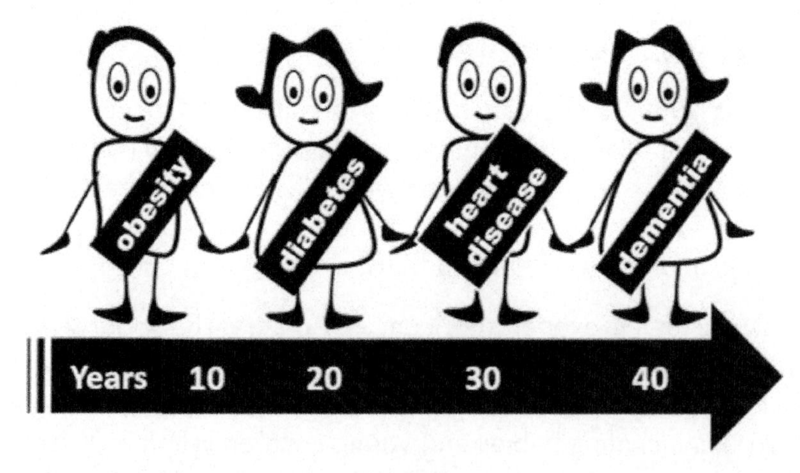

Figure 16. Nutrition-related diseases manifest over many years, often after decades.

The onset of nutrition-related diseases has been insidious, catching people unaware, not linking processed foods with added sugar content in all its varieties as the real cause of the sorry state of affairs.

> 'Saturated fat and cholesterol in the diet are not the cause of coronary heart disease. That myth is the greatest scientific deception of this century, perhaps of any century. One day the true cause of coronary heart disease will be found and the disorder will be prevented. When that happens, Keys and his cronies will be exposed.'
>
> *Professor George Mann, Vanderbilt University, 1993*

Getting back to our Fat–Sugar War story, we can only imagine what the outcome for our modern-day society would have been if our anti-sugar activist, John Yudkin and his supporters, had been as combative and ruthless as their opponents, Ancel Keys and his powerful supporters.

Summary

Figure 17 summarises how personalities influenced the outcome of two opposing viewpoints on nutrition and related diseases and how it impacted global business expansions in decades to follow.

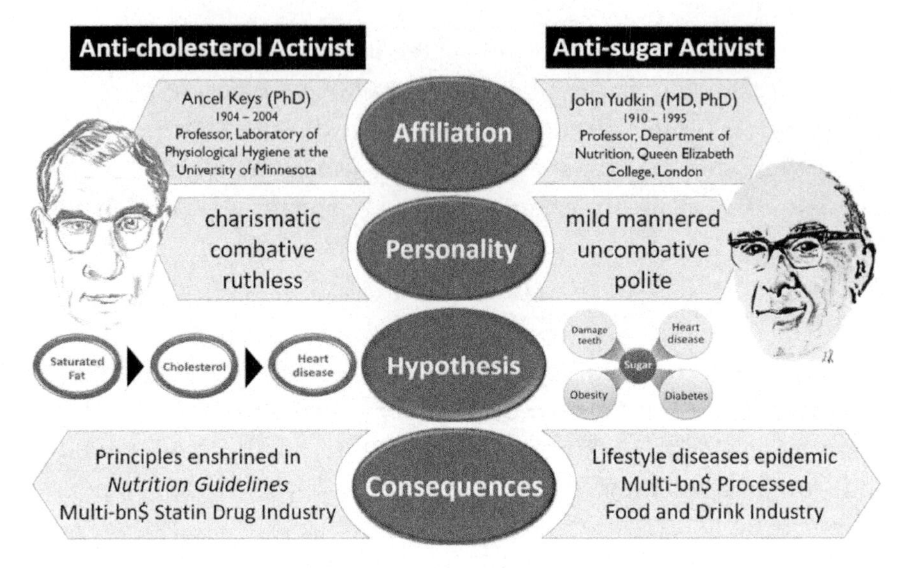

Figure 17. Influence of anti-cholesterol and anti-sugar activists.

Important Points:

- The saturated fat/cholesterol theory of heart disease is false. Saturated fat and cholesterol do not clog your arteries. Our nutritional guidelines are based on this incorrect theory.
- Cholesterol is one of the most vital molecules in the body: without it, we would die.
- If you haven't had a heart attack, taking a cholesterol-lowering statin pill will not prolong your life by one day.
- The dramatic increase in sugar consumption is associated with the rising epidemics of obesity, diabetes, hypertension and heart disease.

Chapter 4

INSULIN RESISTANCE

'When diet is wrong, medicine is of no use.

When diet is correct, medicine is of no need.'

Ancient Ayurvedic Proverb

The Way Sugar is Utilised in our Body

Insulin is the hormone that our body uses to help glucose enter our cells, where it is used by our cell's powerhouse (called the mitochondria) to produce energy. This process ensures that our cells produce enough energy for all the complicated processes they need to sustain and support optimal health. If insulin doesn't do its job properly – when it can no longer open the cell door for glucose to enter – we call this condition insulin resistance. This means that the affected cells and tissues can no longer perform their normal functions for a lack of energy. For those interested in a detailed description of the discovery of the insulin resistance syndrome and its medical ramifications, I recommend reading Prof Tim Noakes' blog series: *CrossFit: It's the Insulin Resistance, Stupid: Parts 1–11.*

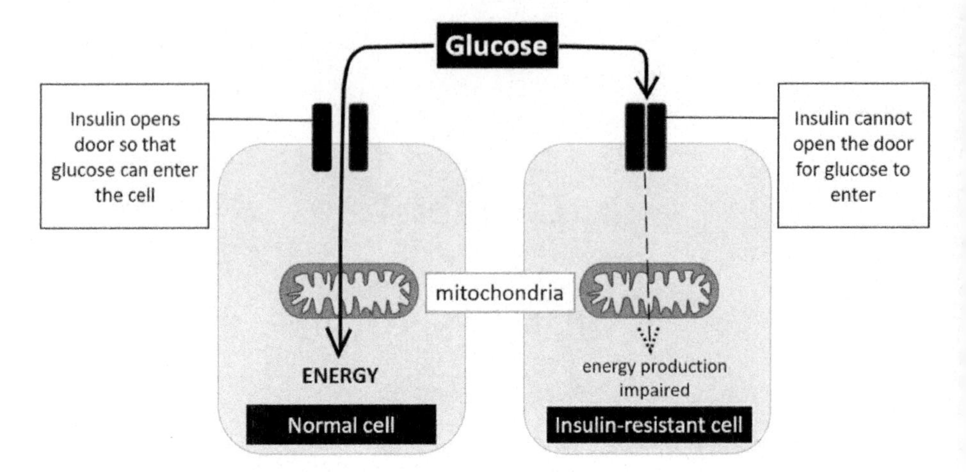

Figure 18. Energy production: a normal cell vs an insulin-resistant cell.

Insulin resistance is not something that happens suddenly; it is a condition that develops over years to decades and progressively worsens with time as tissues become more and more resistant or insensitive to the action of insulin. As a result, insulin must be secreted in increasingly greater amounts and is the hallmark of this disease: very high insulin levels in the blood. When high insulin levels are present for extended periods (years to decades), it leads to the development of diseases that doctors have considered in the past as completely different conditions. All these symptoms can now be traced back to the same cause, i.e. *insulin resistance*. The way the disease manifests itself depends on the organ or organs most affected.

For example, if the disease of insulin resistance manifests in the muscles it is called 'diabetes', in our livers it is called 'fatty liver disease', in our brains it is called 'dementia' and in the ovaries of women, 'polycystic ovary syndrome'.

We now know that insulin resistance is the forerunner of almost all the non-infectious, chronic medical conditions that currently plague modern humans: from Alzheimer's disease or dementia to hypertension, type 2 diabetes, polycystic ovarian syndrome, coronary heart disease and even cancer, to name a few.

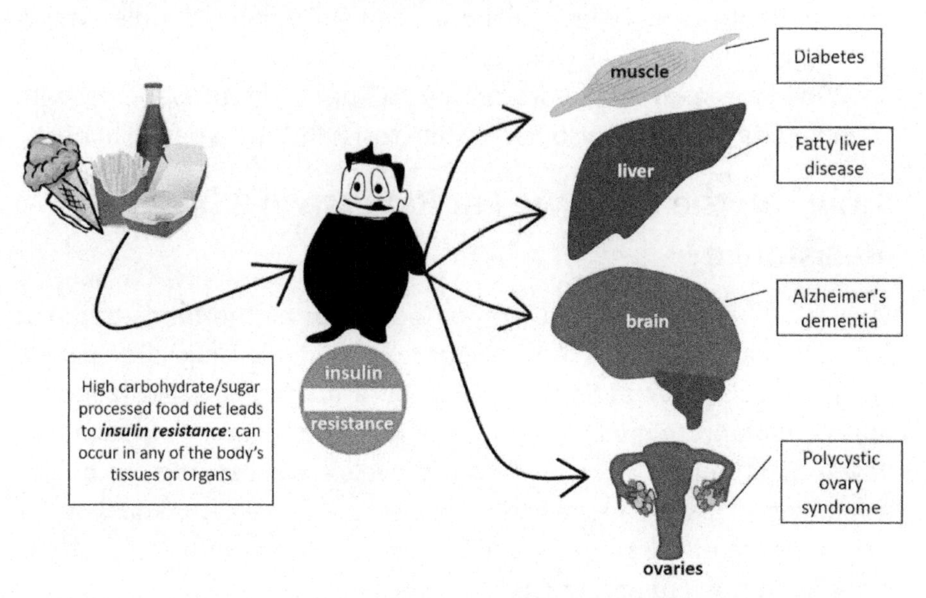

Figure 19. Insulin resistance in different organs leads to different symptoms and/or diseases.

Unfortunately, doctors are not trained to test their patient's insulin levels, and the condition is, therefore, hardly ever diagnosed. This is the unfortunate reality since medical students are taught the incorrect fat–cholesterol theory of heart disease at medical school, instead of the real culprit (carbs/sugar) of modern-day lifestyle diseases. If insulin resistance is diagnosed in a timely fashion, the condition can be corrected and reversed by simple and correct dietary advice. If left alone, it will progress to manifest symptoms in a great many people in one or more target organs affected.

Most patients are unaware that they are ***insulin resistant***

It is not possible to predict who will develop one or more of these diseases. For example, in 1999 scientists from Rotterdam reported that patients with type 2 diabetes had an almost double risk of developing dementia as well. In another study, published in Diabetes in 2004, researchers reported that 80 per cent of patients with Alzheimer's dementia also had insulin resistance or type 2 diabetes.

How can the Food we Eat Reverse Insulin Resistance?

As we can see from the illustration below, of all the foodstuffs that we eat, carbohydrates are responsible for releasing the highest insulin levels after eating, followed by a medium insulin response after eating protein while fat has the lowest impact on blood insulin levels. Remember, when high insulin levels are present in our bodies for long periods, we first develop insulin resistance often followed by one or more of the target organ diseases. It is, therefore, something we should prevent at all costs!

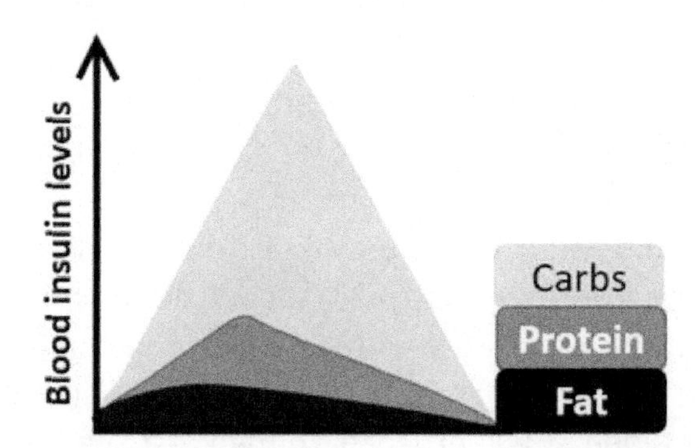

Figure 20. Difference in the amount of insulin released after eating carbohydrates, protein or fat.

It stands to reason then that we need to be very careful about our level of carbohydrate consumption! The food and drink industry provides us with thousands of processed food and drink products packed with carbohydrates (including sugar). People who are consuming any of these products regularly should be warned about the possibility that they may already suffer from insulin resistance – unaware and undiagnosed – especially if they don't have any symptoms.

Our Fat Stores

For most people, the thought of our body's fat stores is not a pleasant one. It is something we think that we can do without, especially if we suffer from an ever-expanding waistline. But this is not the case, our fat stores are very important. In days gone by, as stated earlier in the book, our ancestors relied heavily on their fat stores during times when food was scarce or during a famine. Our bodies have been programmed through millions of years of evolution to switch to a different energy source when its glucose supply runs low. It starts to utilise fat for energy. This is a natural process; in fact, it is the way our body's metabolism has been programmed. There is one hormone above all that is very important in controlling the process of fat storage and fat depletion. Yes, you guessed correctly. It is *insulin*.

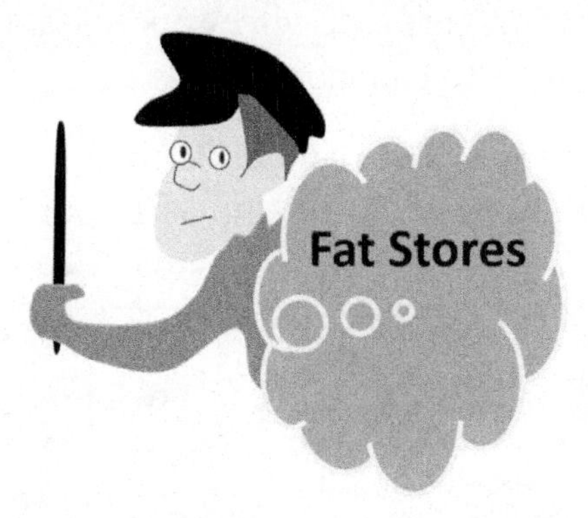

Figure 21. Insulin is the fat-storage hormone and protects our fat stores from being utilised.

Here is how it works: when we have a steady supply of glucose, insulin levels rise, which then allows glucose to enter our cells for energy production. When that process is completed, all *excess energy* (not needed by our cells) is now stored as fat (the reserve energy storage system for our bodies). As mentioned before, insulin is called the *fat-storage hormone*. The key message here is that the higher our insulin levels the greater the amount of fat storage whilst low insulin levels open the fat storage gate so that fat can be utilised as an energy fuel.

High insulin levels = **Expanding** fat stores
Low insulin levels = **Shrinking** fat stores

Another key point is that the body cannot use both energy fuels at the same time, i.e. glucose and fat. Of the two fuel types, glucose is dominant, meaning that if there is an external supply of glucose (eating), only glucose will be utilised for energy, while the fat stores are left intact or expanding, depending on the amount of glucose supplied and level of insulin released. In other words, if you eat a lot of carbohydrates, high insulin levels will be released and fat storage is the result. If we continue doing this week in, week out, month in, month out, we gain weight, develop insulin resistance, eventually become overweight or even obese, while remaining hungry and feeling fatigued. The process is driven by our metabolism and the only way to turn it around is to change *what we eat*.

The way to do this is to cut right back on the amount of glucose (carbohydrates and sugar) that we eat. When our body senses that

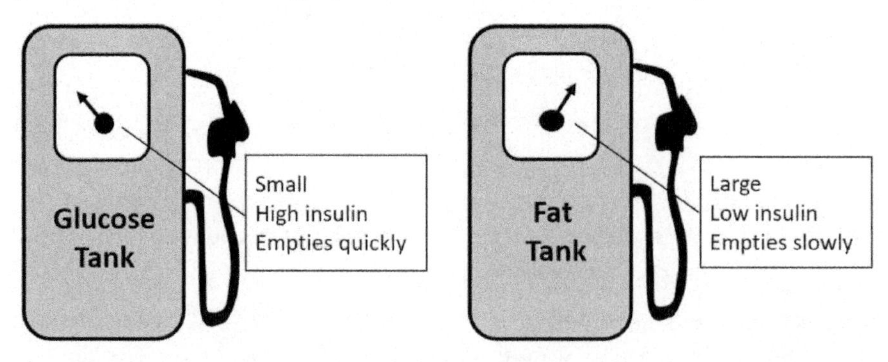

Figure 22. Our body has two fuel tanks: a small glucose and a large fat tank.

the glucose supply is low and that the release of insulin has *dramatically dropped* because of it, it opens up the fat storage gate to access our reserve energy storage system!

Our fat tank (running on low insulin levels) is much larger than our glucose energy tank; therefore, it is the healthiest energy source for our bodies. To keep it that way, keep your carb supply (intake) low. That way you will be able to control your weight and stop the fat storage/weight gaining process.

That brings us to one of the false dogmas of nutrition: Eating fat makes you fat. Just as we have seen that the saturated fat/cholesterol theory of heart disease is not true, so the link between fat consumption and obesity is absolute nonsense. It is the anti-fat pro-sugar lobby that is relentlessly repeating this misinformation, enslaving millions of people around the globe on this roller-coaster ride of high-carb-weight-gain-then-yo-yo-dieting-going-nowhere routine.

Eating fat doesn't make you fat
Eating carbs and sugar makes you fat

Ketones or ketone bodies are the fuel that our fat stores produce. Ketones are normally produced in our bodies when we maintain a low carb intake. Some people get very uncomfortable when ketones are mentioned because they link it to the medical condition of 'diabetic ketoacidosis'. This condition happens when the disease of type 1 or type 2 diabetics is out of control and massive amounts of ketones are produced. This is a dangerous condition with ketone levels ten-fold higher than nutritional ketosis. As Jeff Volek and Stephen Phinney mention in their book *The Art and Science of Low Carbohydrate Living*, it is like the difference between a gentle rain and a torrential downpour!

How do we get Enough Glucose on a Low Carb Diet?

The brain needs a portion of its fuel to come from glucose. The glucose amount it needs can easily be produced by the liver from fat and protein that we eat. The process is called *gluconeogenesis*. There is, therefore, no need for us to eat a lot of extra glucose in our diet to ensure that our brains get enough fuel!

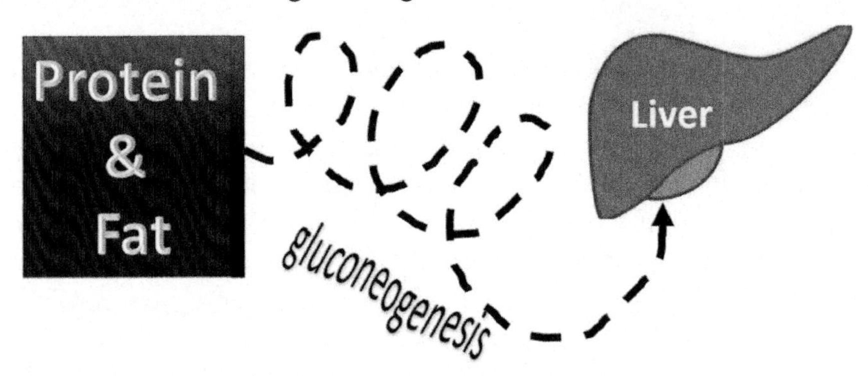

Figure 23. Our body makes glucose from fat and protein through a process called gluconeogenesis.

Important Points:

- Dietary fat has the least impact on raising insulin levels, while carbohydrate (sugar and starch) intake is associated with the highest insulin response.
- Insulin resistance is the most common metabolic disorder that people suffer from today.
- Insulin resistance in different organs leads to different symptoms and/or diseases.
- Insulin is the 'fat storage' hormone.

Chapter 5

DIETARY DISEASES

'Health is not valued until sickness comes.'

Thomas Fuller

Diabetes

We are talking about type 2 diabetes in this section, the type of diabetes that is caused by the food we eat. In the previous chapter, we explained how the disease process starts – *insulin resistance* – which often progresses into full-blown type 2 diabetes, which is usually diagnosed when the GP orders a blood test that shows that the blood sugar values are very high. Most of these patients are also overweight or obese, and may already, or will in the future, have one or more of the other lifestyle diseases such as high blood pressure, infertility, dementia, etc.

The typical response from the GP after diagnosing diabetes is to put the patient immediately on anti-diabetic medication. This starts a lifelong journey of medical treatment for the patient with increased dosages and often several types of diabetic drugs being added to try to control the condition as the years march on. Ultimately, even insulin injections are offered to try to slow down the relentless disease progression. This sequence of events cannot and will never address the underlying condition.

The tragedy is that the diet of the patient is often *not discussed*. Neither the patient nor, even more tragically, the doctor, is aware that the basic underlying cause of the condition is that the patient's carbohydrate intake is *too high* for the body to cope. Their blood insulin and glucose levels are both high, but their body's tissues are no longer responsive to insulin and, therefore, glucose can no longer efficiently get into their cells.

Think about this – if you have a gluten or peanut intolerance, would you ingest gluten or peanuts? Of course not, you would avoid it at all costs! The same logic applies to diabetes. For example – eating a potato (starch) can raise your blood sugar as much as eating nine teaspoons of sugar! If instead, you avoid sugar and starch, it will result in lower blood glucose levels and, as a result of that, lower insulin levels, which again, in time, will reduce or eliminate your need for medication. *It is that simple!* By *changing your diet*, you can effectively reverse many of the negative effects associated with diabetes.

Choosing foods low in carbohydrates is a safe and easy way to help you control your blood sugar. Review the table on the next page – you may be surprised to see the amount of sugar equivalents in the different kinds of foods. The food types high in teaspoon sugar values are the ones to be avoided.

Research shows that low-carbohydrate diets are a safe and effective option for treating and reversing type 2 diabetes as demonstrated by the following examples:

- In 2019, the American Diabetes Association (ADA) stated that reducing carbohydrate intake was the most effective nutritional strategy for improving blood sugar control in patients with diabetes.

Food Item	Glycaemic index	Serve size g	How does each food affect blood glucose compared with one 4g teaspoon of table sugar?
Basmati rice	69	150	10.1
Potato, white, boiled	96	150	9.1
French Fries baked	64	150	7.5
Spaghetti White boiled	39	180	6.6
Sweet corn boiled	60	80	4.0
Frozen peas, boiled	51	80	1.3
Banana	62	120	5.7
Apple	39	120	2.3
Wholemeal Small slice	74	30	3.0
Broccoli	15	80	0.2
Eggs	0	60	0

Other foods in the very low glycaemic range would be chicken, oily fish, almonds, mushrooms, cheese, meat

Figure 24. Teaspoon sugar equivalents for food items.

Source: Dr David Unwin's NICE Endorsed Sugar Equivalence Infographics, ©Public Health Collaboration.

- Virta Health published a study in 2019 of 349 people with type 2 diabetes who either followed a very-low-carb diet or a standard diet. After one year, 97 per cent of those in the low-carb group had reduced or stopped their insulin use, while 58 per cent were no longer diagnosed as having diabetes (disease in remission), while in the standard diet group there was no change.
- In England, Dr David Unwin, of Norwood Surgery in Southport, is a strong advocate of lifestyle medicine. He won the National Health Service (NHS) Innovator of the Year Award in 2016. At the Public Health Conference in 2020, he reported that of the 300 patients with diabetes he had treated so far, 47 per cent achieved drug-free type 2 diabetes remission. That represented an annual saving of £50,000 for NHS England, and a potential saving of £266 million if all the practices in England implemented a similar protocol!

Low-carb Diets are not New

William Banting (1796–1878)
London undertaker. Published his *"Letter on Corpulence, Addressed to the Public"* in 1862, describing how he won his battle against obesity by adopting an eating plan avoiding starchy food with generous amounts of protein and fat.

Dr Wilhelm Ebstein (1836–1912)
Medical doctor and Professor at the University of Göttingen, Germany. An early proponent of the low-carb, high-fat diet for treating diabetes, gout and obesity. He forbade the eating of sugar, sweets of all kinds and potatoes in every form.

Dr Robert Atkins (1930–2003)
New York physician. Treated thousands of patients for obesity and related diseases by advising them to eat meat not maize and saturated fat not grains.

Figure 25. Low-carb diets are not new.

When people with type 2 diabetes embark on lowering their carbohydrate intake, they often notice that even on the first day of the diet their blood sugar levels improve (lower glucose values). It is essential for patients to have their own blood sugar monitoring device at home since their need for medications, especially insulin, is dramatically reduced. As they continue on this nutrition programme, substantial weight loss often follows and, generally, people feel much better, have more energy and alertness, and many of their other health markers will improve, including a lowering of their blood pressure.

It is very important for people with diabetes who want to make changes to their lifestyle to inform their GP in advance and work very closely with him or her on making treatment dosage adjustments. If your health care provider is not enthusiastic about helping you pursue a natural solution to reverse or improve your diabetes, try to find one who is able and willing to help.

Even today, many health professionals cannot accept that their beliefs regarding nutrition are not based on sound scientific data. This has led to several trials and personal prosecutions over the years. In 2014, Professor Tim Noakes was taken to trial by the Health

Professionals Council in South Africa (HPCSA) for promoting a low-carb, high-fat diet on social media and, in 2016, Dr Gary Fettke, an orthopaedic surgeon, was sanctioned by the Australian Health Practitioners Regulation Agency (AHPRA) for recommending a low-carb lifestyle to his patients with diabetes. Two years later, in 2018, the AHPRA repealed its decision in its entirety.

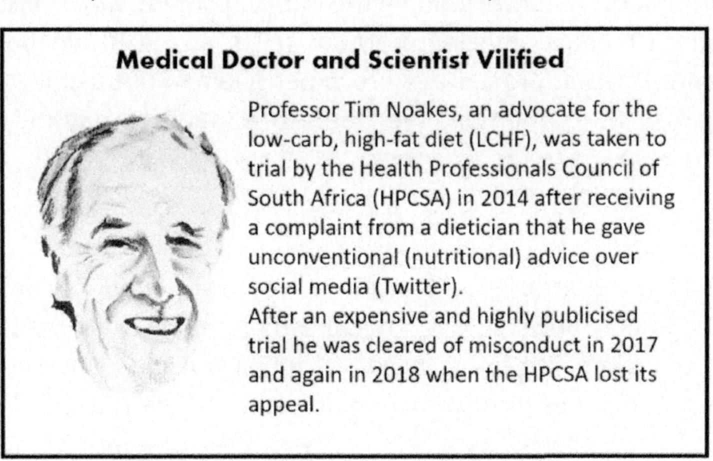

Figure 26. Medical doctor and scientist vilified.

What is TOFI?

Tofi stands for '**T**hin **O**utside, **F**at **I**nside'. In short, it is someone who doesn't seem to carry excess weight because their fat is hidden in their abdominal area around their internal organs. They appear to be healthy, but are, in fact, at high risk of developing one or more of the lifestyle diseases (heart disease, type 2 diabetes and other diseases associated with insulin resistance). Some people use the term 'thin diabetic' to describe this condition.

The condition was first described in 1981 by Ruderman et al., identifying a subgroup of normal-weight individuals with all the characteristics of insulin resistance. Typically, they have high blood sugar, high insulin values, high levels of blood triglycerides and often high blood pressure, all of this despite having a body mass index (BMI) < 25 kg/m2.

Despite the outward appearance of being 'thin', the underlying metabolic process (insulin resistance) is exactly the same as seen in people presenting with excess weight or obesity. The increased amount of fat tissue surrounding the internal organs can be visualised by modern medical imaging methods (CT scans, MRI or abdominal ultrasound). These procedures are expensive and not usually utilised to diagnose this condition. We, therefore, need to rely on regular blood tests to make the diagnosis.

Cancer

Cancer or malignancy, is called a disease of 'civilisation' or a 'Western disease', mainly because it is not something that archaeologists have found in ancient hunter-gatherer societies nor was it described in traditional societies prior to the colonisation of the Americas, Africa, Asia and Australia by European settlers (see Chapter 3). Western diseases were, therefore, uncommon in indigenous populations isolated from Western influence.

Cancer is a Modern Disease

In 1915, Frederick Hoffman, chief statistician for the Prudential Insurance Company of America, published an eight-hundred-plus-page report, *Mortality from Cancer Throughout the World*. It concluded that a large number of medical missionaries and other trained medical observers, living for years among native races throughout the world, found that cancer mortality was 'extremely rare among North American Indians and the primitive races of Asia and Africa'. Hugh Trowell and Denis Burkitt, two British missionary physicians who worked in East Africa before, during and after the Second World War, compiled a list of Western diseases from hospital surveys from five continents. They observed how the spectrum of disease of indigenous populations changed over time as they adapted to Western diets and urban lifestyles.

A Growing Epidemic

Cancer is now predicted to overtake heart disease as the leading cause of death in Western societies. Breast cancer incidence has more than doubled in the last 50 years and, in the US, breast cancer now accounts for 30 per cent of all female cancers. Failure to manage the development of cancers effectively is, in a large part, due to our misunderstanding of the origin of cancer.

Is Cancer a Genetic Disease?

The traditional medical view is that cancer is a genetic disease. The discovery of millions of gene changes over the years in different cancers has led to the perception that cancer is not a single disease, but a collection of many different diseases. The thinking is that these genetic changes (mutations) that occur in the nucleus of cells drive abnormal growth of the affected cells, which eventually results in the development of cancer.

But is it?

More recent research has shown that cancer can also occur in the absence of gene mutations. Another interesting fact is that, although humans and chimpanzees are genetically 98.5 per cent identical, breast cancer has never been documented in chimps, suggesting that diet and lifestyle issues, rather than genetic mutations may be a key component in the development of this disease.

Further support that cancer is not primarily a genetic disease comes from cell nucleus transfer experiments. In these experiments, the cell nucleus, which contains the genetic material of the cell, is transferred between cancer and normal cells. Several researchers have shown that when the nucleus of a cancer cell containing mutations is 'transplanted' into a normal cell, these hybrid cells will produce *normal cells*. The opposite happens when the nucleus of a normal cell (with no mutations) is transplanted into a cancer cell since this hybrid cell will then produce more *cancer cells*. The conclusion from this experiment is that it is not the genetic material in the nucleus of the cancer cell per se that contributes to the process, but something that happens in the rest of the cell – i.e. in the cytoplasm of the cell where all the metabolic processes take place.

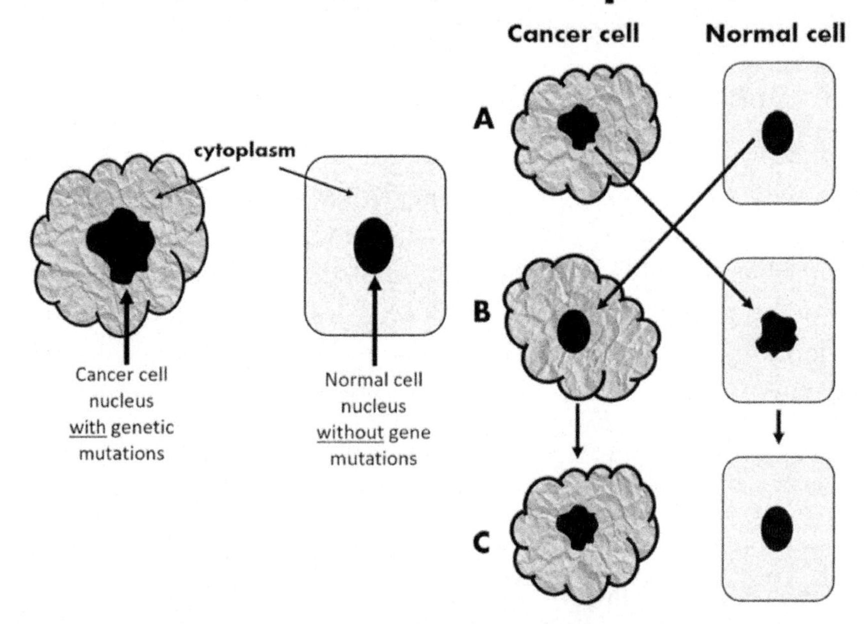

Figure 27. Cell nucleus transfer experiments.

(A) Cancer cell with an abnormal nucleus and a normal cell with a normal nucleus; (B) Cancer cell nucleus transferred into a normal cell and a normal cell nucleus transferred into a cancer cell; (C) Cancer cell with normal nucleus results in more cancer cells, while a normal cell with a cancer cell nucleus results in more normal cells.

Redrawn from Seyfried et al., Cancer as a metabolic disease: Implications for novel therapies. *Carcinogenesis*, 2014.

How are Cancer Cells Different?

We cannot discuss malignancy without considering cancer cells and what is driving them to behave like rogues, no longer adhering to the 'law of the land' or in biology language, metabolic cellular control.

Normally, healthy cells in our body have strict control systems in place to stop unlimited cell division or proliferation. Cancer cells, on the other hand, don't adhere to these control systems, often as a result of genetic mutations. These mutations can change the operation of metabolic pathways in cancer cells, making them more sensitive to certain nutrients that fuel cell growth.

It is All About Sugar (Glucose)

The dramatic increase in cancer, such as breast cancer, is possibly due to increased oestrogen exposure through eating highly processed food, containing high carbohydrate levels, that we have been exposed to over the past four decades.

Sugar or glucose is the nutrient of prime importance to cancer cells. In fact, cancer cells use glucose differently from normal cells. To understand how cancer cells operate, let's first look at the process in normal cells. Here, glucose is used in the presence of oxygen to produce a large amount of energy (adenosine triphosphate or ATP) utilizing the cell's own powerhouse, called the mitochondria. Cells need energy to process all the complicated cellular processes required for us to live a healthy life. If oxygen isn't available to body cells, anaerobic (without oxygen) metabolism kicks in to produce energy (a much less efficient process) and lactic acid is formed as a by-product. Lactate build-up in the body is associated with serious diseases such as sepsis, cardiac arrest, seizures, etc.

In contrast, cancer cells use glucose in the presence of oxygen to form large amounts of lactic acid and, in this process, they bypass the cell's powerhouse (mitochondria). It appears that the mitochondria in cancer cells are structurally defective, which can be observed under the electron microscope. This process was first described in the 1920s by the German biochemist and medical doctor, Otto Warburg. Warburg was a great friend of Albert Einstein and his striking discovery earned him the Nobel prize for Physiology and Medicine in 1931.

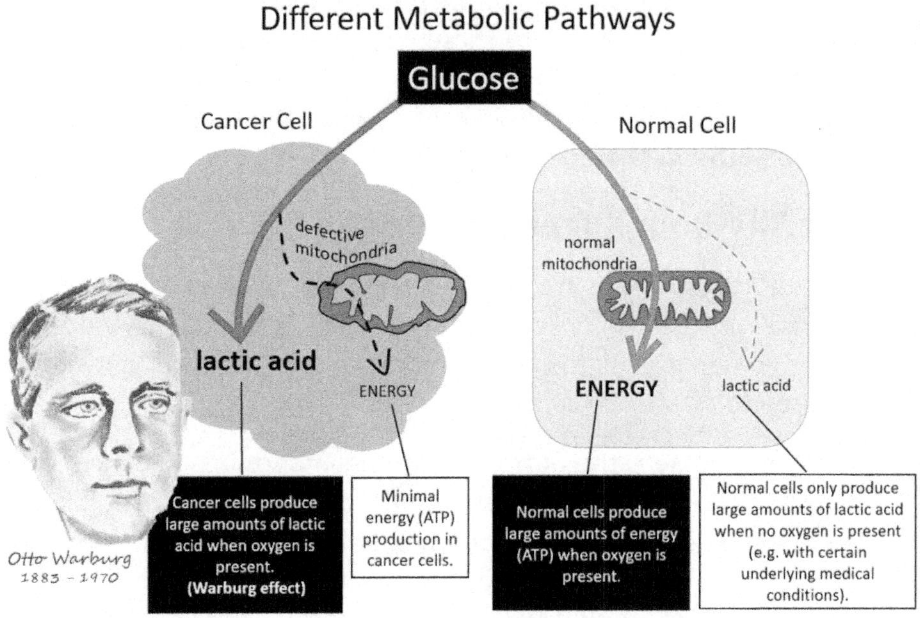

Figure 28. Cancer cells and normal cells handle glucose very differently.

Cancer researchers today acknowledge the importance of the Warburg effect in cancer development and now link not only glucose but also the amino acid glutamine as the most important sources of fuel for cancer cells. It is a well-known fact that high levels of blood glucose accelerate cancer cell growth, and should be avoided. A recent Norwegian study published in *BMC Cancer* (2019) showed that breast cancer patients, who received glucose before surgery, had a higher rate of cancer recurrence and worse survival rate than the control group that didn't receive glucose. It seems that over time cancer cells become more and more dependent on glucose and more vulnerable to glucose deprivation.

This is not a new fact. As far back as 1921, the biochemist Alexander Braunstein noted that glucose disappeared from the urine of patients with diabetes after they were diagnosed with cancer, suggesting that glucose was used by the cancer or cancer cells as a fuel!

This dependency of cancer cells on glucose can be used to detect malignancy in the body. The method used, consists of injecting radioactive glucose into the body, and then, by using a special scan, determines where the glucose is concentrated and utilised. This type of scan is called fluorodeoxyglucose-positron emission tomography or FDG-PET.

Hungry Cancer Cells Consume Their Host

Another example of how cancer cells depend on glucose as a fuel is the fact that extreme weight loss or cachexia is a common manifestation of terminal cancer. We have already described how cancer cells alter metabolic processes in the body. As part of the cancer process, the cancer cells release inflammation molecules (called cytokines) that influence other tissues and organs directly. These cytokines, for instance, drive the process of forming new glucose molecules in the liver through a process called *gluconeogenesis* (literally meaning forming new glucose).

The liver obtains the building blocks to form glucose by recycling lactic acid which is produced in large amounts by the cancer cells. As the cancer develops and grows, the demand or hunger for glucose expands, so other sources of glucose fuel must be found. Two other sources feed this demand: protein from breaking down muscle tissue and fatty acids from breaking down the fat stores (a process called *lipolysis*). These processes lead to progressive muscle wasting and loss of fat, which are the two hallmarks of cancer cachexia. At the same time, more glucose is made available for the ever-greater need of the expanding cancer cell mass.

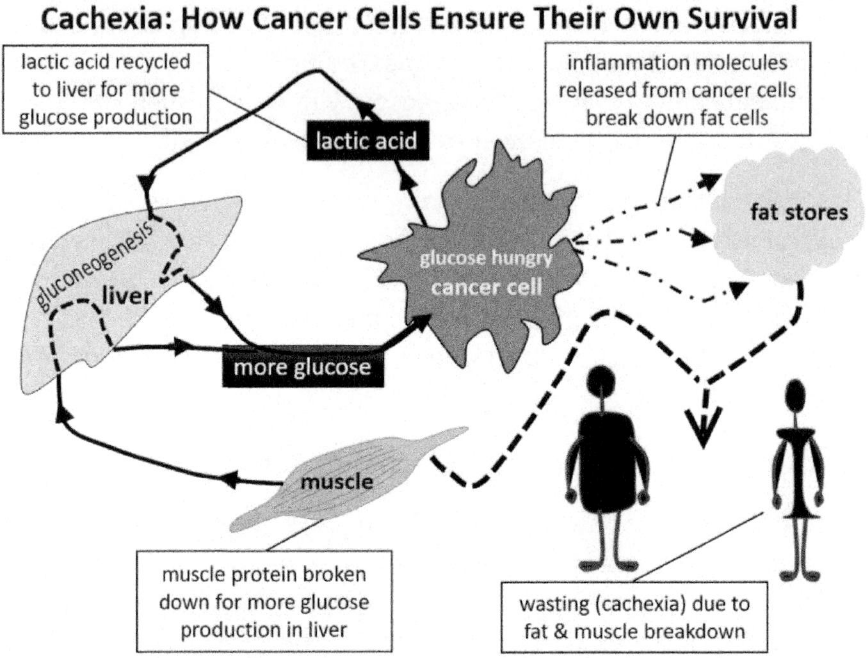

Figure 29. Cachexia: How cancer cells ensure their own survival.

Based on: Klement & Kämmerer, Is there a role for carbohydrate restriction in the treatment and prevention of cancer? *Nutrition & Metabolism*, 2011.

How can Diet Help?

With this in mind, dietary intervention in addition to regular cancer therapy is becoming a logical and additional strategy for managing cancer patients. This therapy focuses on lowering the amount of carbohydrates that cancer patients eat. The reason for this is that all carbohydrates ingested are broken down into glucose molecules by the body's metabolic processes and, as we have seen, glucose is the food that feeds cancer cells. A low-carbohydrate diet in the context of cancer therapy, also called 'ketogenic metabolic therapy' is based on the principle that if glucose is not available for energy, the body will switch to using fat as a fuel source. The breakdown products from fat are called ketones, hence the name 'ketogenic' to describe this type of dietary therapy.

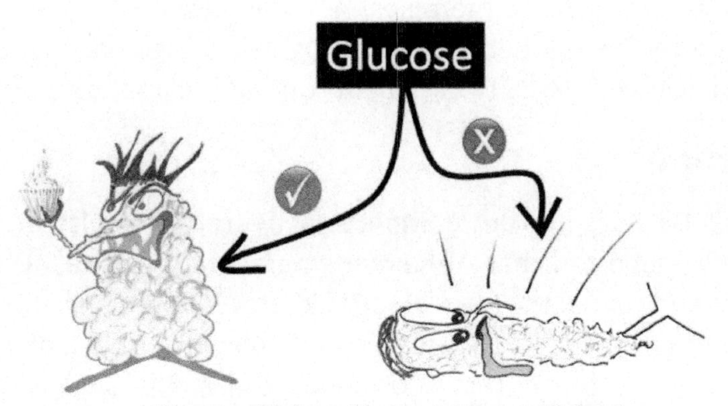

Glucose withdrawal induces cancer cell death

The utilisation of fat fuel (ketones) by cells, as a natural fuel source, has been known for over a hundred years. Cancer cells cannot use ketones for fuel and, hence, they cannot survive and will die as long as the cancer patient maintains low levels of carbohydrate/glucose intake. This fact greatly assists and augments the effectiveness of other cancer therapies received by cancer patients and offers a complementary strategy to standard cancer therapy. Carb restriction not only affects the primary cancer but also restricts the spread of cancer cells and inflammation associated with chemotherapy. It has also been shown that a low-carb diet reduces the risk of a recurrence of breast cancer and results in an increased overall survival rate for breast cancer and other cancer patients.

Many studies have now shown the safety and feasibility of cancer patients tolerating a low-carb/keto diet, and oncologists and other health care providers should consider combining this dietary approach with standard care modalities, such as chemotherapy and radiation. If the cancer support team is unwilling to entertain such an approach, it may be very worthwhile for patients to seek alternative providers who are more familiar with this approach.

Another fascinating finding is that the anti-diabetic drug, Metformin, used to lower blood glucose in patients with type 2 diabetes, seems to prevent malignancy as well as provide improved outcomes when used with other cancer therapies. A study published in *The BMJ* in 2005, showed that patients on this drug have a significantly reduced risk of cancer compared with patients on other diabetic medications.

Dementia

In 2005, Dr Suzanne de la Monte, a neuropathologist at Brown University, reported that Alzheimer's dementia (AD) was a form of diabetes and coined the term type 3 diabetes. Another way to explain it is that Alzheimer's is diabetes of the brain while type 2 diabetes is diabetes of the body. This information came as a surprise to the medical community who thought dementia was an unrelated brain disease and not a metabolic disorder. Many patients and their physicians still regard dementia as a mysterious and inevitable disease without any meaningful treatment.

AD consists of two forms; early-onset AD (or familial AD) constitutes less than 5 per cent of all AD cases and is normally diagnosed before the age of 65 years, while late-onset AD is the most common cause accounting for 60 to 80 per cent of all dementia cases. But what if the most common or garden variety dementia is largely preventable and disease progression can be altered by lifestyle choices?

Sounds too good to be true?

Brain changes begin decades before there are any clinical manifestations of dementia. Typically, the first brain areas affected by dementia are the areas where learning and memory functions are based (medial temporal and orbitofrontal regions of the brain), and the disease then spreads progressively to other brain areas. Clinically, the disease starts with progressive memory loss and a gradual decline in cognitive function, eventually leading to premature death, which occurs, typically, three to nine years after diagnosis.

The rate of AD increases sharply over the age of 50 and is very common in overweight, obese and diabetic patients. In 2013, Gudala et al., published a meta-analysis of 28 studies which showed a 73 per cent increased risk of dementia in patients with diabetes. Dementia Statistics Hub (www.dementiastatistics.org) predicts that globally the number of people living with dementia will increase from 50 million in 2018 to 152 million in 2050, a *204 per cent increase*.

New Name for Alzheimer's Disease: Type 3 Diabetes

Researchers have shown that the brain tissue of patients with AD show similar biochemical and microscopic changes to those patients with diabetes. Their brains typically show insulin resistance, inflammation, abnormal glucose and energy metabolism. With insulin resistance, not enough glucose can enter the brain cells to produce the energy needed for normal brain cell functions.

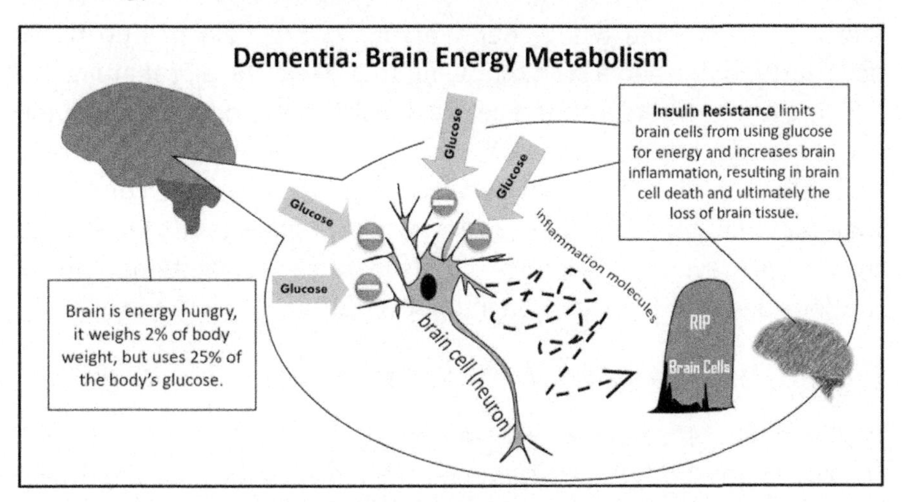

Figure 30. Dementia: Brain energy metabolism.

Prolonged insulin resistance can result in brain cell death affecting memory, thinking, judgement, reasoning and perception.

Ultimately this leads to brain cell death, which is further enhanced by the release of multiple inflammation molecules (cytokines) that further impact the brain cells and supporting tissues, resulting in more damage and further loss of brain cells and brain tissue.

Mood and Psychiatric Disorders

It is well established that mood and psychiatric disorders, including depression, obsessive-compulsive disorder, bipolar disorder and schizophrenia, are associated with inflammation in the body. Several medical conditions, including obesity, diabetes, cancer, rheumatoid arthritis and multiple sclerosis, are risk factors for depression and bipolar disorder.

There is a very powerful link between the food we eat and the chemicals it releases that impact our brains. For example, we know that man-made oils increase the omega-6 polyunsaturated fats in our body, which have strong inflammatory properties. In 2016, Dr Felice Jacka, an Australian researcher working in the field of nutritional psychiatry, published a study showing that a healthy diet that limited the intake of sweets, refined cereals, fast food, processed food and sugary drinks can improve the mood of people with moderate to severe depression. In the study group, the carbohydrate content of their diet was limited to 37 per cent, which is significantly lower than that of the average Western diet (see Ancient/Traditional versus Modern-day Diet Composition in Chapter 2).

Other Diseases and Conditions

In the previous chapters, we looked at the mechanism of insulin release in the body as well as metabolic drivers of prolonged high levels of insulin. In this chapter, we have discussed several conditions associated with high insulin levels. In 2015, researchers from New Zealand reviewed published data and compiled a much more comprehensive list of diseases and conditions associated with high insulin levels (see Figure 31). In the past, these conditions were not thought of as having a similar metabolic basis, and these findings open up many clinical and research implications. If indeed, our diet underpins the development of these conditions, it should motivate us to make drastic changes in our eating habits. In doing so, we will take a giant step forward in responsibly managing our own health.

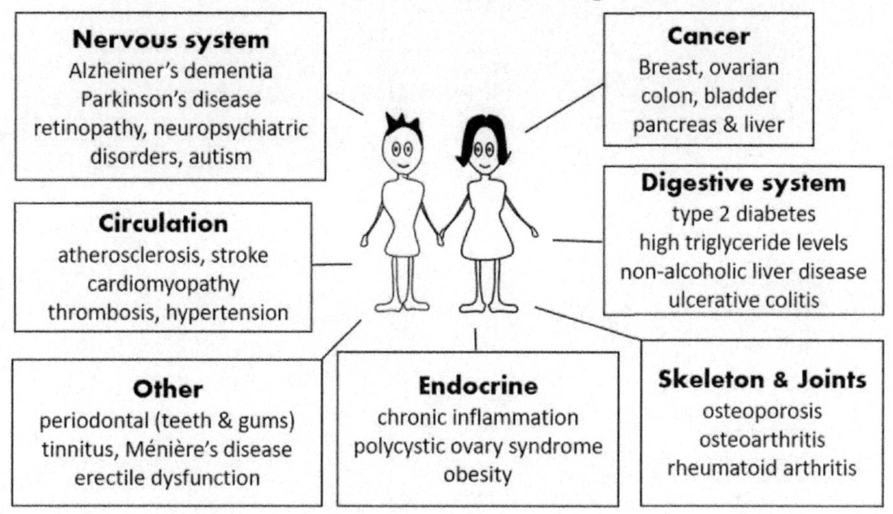

Figure 31. Diseases and conditions linked to high insulin levels.

Based on Crofts C. A. P. et al., Hyperinsulinemia: A unifying theory of chronic disease? *Diabesity* 2015, and Scofield G. et al., *What the Fat?* 2015, p202.

Important Points:

- Type 2 diabetes is a condition related to the body's inability to metabolise glucose. So is dementia and many other conditions.
- Glucose is the most important fuel for cancer cells.
- Carbohydrate restrictive diets have been used for more than two centuries to treat obesity, gout and diabetes. Today, these diets are also used to improve the lot of cancer and dementia sufferers.

Part 2
FOOD PRODUCTION: QUALITY AND QUANTITY

Chapter 6

FARMING METHODS OF THE PAST

'Don't eat anything that your great-great grandmother wouldn't recognise as food.'

Michael Pollan

Have changes in farming methods impacted the quality of the foods we eat today?

Emphatically, in one word, yes!

Memories of My Childhood Farm

I'd like to take you back on a journey to the 1960s when I was growing up on a mixed hill farm in the Scottish Borders. Bear with me here as it is important that you understand the difference in farming methods from then to the present day. It was a typical 1,000-acre hill farm of the time; some crops were grown to provide winter feed for the animals, there was some pastureland for the sheep and the rest was hill farming for sheep and beef cattle. We did have one or two dairy cows – the full-fat milk was just delicious. Full fat was (and still is) king!

My recollection of playing in or running alongside the fields and paddling in the river and the streams brings back memories of a countryside bursting with wildflowers, insects, field mice, butterflies and the sound of bees busily gathering their pollen and, at the same time, pollinating the plants. There was plenty to do if one was fond of nature. This, of course, was before the introduction of pesticides. More on pesticides later.

When we visited the local town to go shopping, we went to the butcher, Mr Waters, who sold beef, lamb, pork and chicken from the surrounding farms, where all the animals romped around in the fields or on the hills and grazed naturally on rich meadow pasture that included clover and buttercups or, in winter, on freshly cropped hay from that year. Yes, there were supplemental feeds for the animals but that was not the norm. Mr Waters knew his stuff and sold us great produce. Every town had a great butcher, unlike now when specialist butchers are becoming increasingly rare. Currently, there is only one UK supermarket chain left which has its own fresh butchery department.

We had a large, highly productive vegetable garden – called in those days a kitchen garden as it was separate from the rest of the garden – which my mother supervised. She was an original 'natural methods' gardener who understood the importance of correct soil nutrients. I remember the barrowloads of manure ('muck' in country language) that was dug into that garden. And, as a result, her vegetables and fruits were delicious. My particular memories include succulent, sweet, mouth-watering strawberries, crisp green lettuce, delicious blackcurrants, tender rhubarb and loads of fresh green veggies. In today's marketplace, all of these fruits and veggies would be called organic. They were, of course, all freshly picked and eaten within hours of picking – the flavours were heavenly. She had green fingers, but I now also understand that she had specific knowledge – correct nutrition for the soil, rotating and cultivating delicious tasty crops.

The same natural methods of crop rotation used by my mother in the kitchen garden were used on the farm to grow the farm crops. As I mentioned above, to protect the soil, crops should ideally be rotated year by year. I distinctly remember asking why some years the crops were grown in certain fields and some fields were pastureland. The answer was simple. As the animals grazed in the meadow pasture, they naturally fertilised the land, thereby partially reinstating the soil's natural nutrients. Often further manure was spread before ploughing and planting the seeds that, over the summer, grew to maturity before harvesting in the autumn. The oats crops I remember were also sown with grass seed so that, after the harvest, the fields could again be used for sheep grazing. And so, the cycle went on, year after year.

If we look at the methods used in 1960s/1970s compared to the present day where farms are farmed more intensively with limited crop rotation, my experience tells me that the previous practices led to tasty nutritious grass-fed meats and delicious homegrown veggies. The taste comparison of foods produced then and now is like the proverbial 'night and day'.

Prior to the 1960s, farmers used organic manure (most farms had plenty if they overwintered any animals) or slag to fertilise their fields. Commercial fertilisers were introduced in the early 1960s and welcomed as being good for improving crop yield.

My memory of poultry is this: hens scratching in the fields close to the hen house and ducks waddling beside the stream foraging happily. And the taste of their eggs was just divine. So much better than even the best organic free-range ones you find today. They were happy hens and ducks and completely comfortable in their glorious environment – the only danger to them being the fox!

In summer, we ate principally fruit and veggies grown from the garden, and, in winter, we bought seasonal fruit and vegetables from the local fruit and veg shop. All this was before the advent of the supermarket – little did we realise when convenience shopping arrived that it would be the first step towards our downward health spiral. This, taken in conjunction with changes in farming methods, food production methods and government food guidelines, has led to the explosion of lifestyle diseases today: diabetes, obesity, cancer and dementia. The rot had set in.

There was an abundance of fresh fish. On our doorstep, there was a clean free-flowing unpolluted river, one of the tributaries of the world-famous salmon fishing river (the Tweed), which then had a good stock of healthy trout and salmon. Each week, a fishmonger from the East Coast of Scotland travelled up the valley bringing his supplies of freshly caught North Sea fish. He stopped at every farm – those were the days! Salmon was only fished by permit but we did have an industrious farm cat who used to hook the occasional salmon from a stream swollen by floodwater and drag it home. She was a great scavenger and used to leave several offerings at the back door – the salmon was definitely the best! And it was delicious freshly poached – very different from today's flaccid farmed fish option.

So, is Everything in the Garden Still as Rosy?

Er, not exactly! Let's look at some current methods, lest we think that farming today is the same as in previous decades. First, we must also acknowledge that marketing expertise has developed into an art. We see glamorous marketing materials showing happy cows in green pastures, lambs running and gambolling in the fields, etc. and imagine that is the source of the product we are buying. Regrettably not – it's all imagery and how, in particular, it makes us feel. Do bear in mind that the Food Industry = Big Money. So, their marketing experts can create a picture of health, happiness and feel-good factor by showing a picture of a farmyard chicken scratching merrily when the reality is far from that. The poultry industry, alongside other animal husbandry methods, has been replaced by highly specialised (and profitable) businesses. The term 'factory farm' originated when chickens were found to be so much more profitable if they were reared and housed inside in their thousands rather than foraging merrily in the farmyard. And poultry is not the only area of specialisation. Sheep, cattle, pigs, fish – the list is endless. More of this to follow on future pages.

You may recollect that I described my experiences of running through fields teeming with wildlife. Why are those same fields now, by comparison, almost devoid of life?

Since 1990, the Pesticide Action Network UK reports that crops are more exposed to toxic pesticides than ever. The amount of land treated with pesticides has increased by 63 per cent. This has serious harmful effects on our environment – farmland bird species continue to decline, bees and pollinators are being poisoned, water sources are being contaminated and also, worryingly, pesticides are present in the food we eat.

It is also so apt that, today, as I am writing this chapter, the UK National Farmers' Union (NFU) is asking us to sign a petition to ensure that the food we eat in our homes, schools, hospitals and restaurants or buy from shops in the UK matches the high standards of production expected of UK farmers. At the time of writing, COVID-19 has particularly highlighted the importance of food security and traceability. This also has relevance for householders in the UK as this year the government is negotiating trade deals (including food) with many countries whose food production methods are currently illegal here.

Chapter 7

PROCESSED FOODS AND INDUSTRIAL FARMING

'The food you eat can either be the safest and most powerful form of medicine – or the slowest form of poison.'

Ann Wigmore

What do we know and should we care?

Processed Foods

Processed foods and ready-made meals are the norm globally in 2020, and we really need to educate ourselves as to their content and quality if we are to drive forward a health campaign for optimal health for ourselves.

The NHS in the UK describes processed foods as being not just microwave meals and ready meals but any food that has been altered in some way during preparation. This includes such basic methods as freezing, canning and baking. Common processed foods include breakfast cereals, tinned vegetables, bread, snacks such as crisps/chips, cakes and biscuits and soft drinks/sodas as well as vegetable oils.

I thought I understood that but had to seriously ask myself the question: 'How much do I understand or know about processed food?' And the honest answer was: 'Not much!' I knew it was certainly the 'go-to' food that sits tantalisingly on supermarket shelves in easy-to-purchase cartons, packets or bottles. Check it out for yourself the next time you are at the supermarket and see which products are directly in line with your eye. It's quite revealing! Another aspect I certainly didn't think about was how long a shelf life the product had and the implications of that, i.e. what made the product last so long. As a normal working mum, I only thought in terms of convenience purchasing or that it would save me time in the kitchen when I returned home tired from work and needed to prepare a meal.

It took a health scare to really bring me to my senses. What was I eating, what were the ingredients/contents, why had my health gone on a downward spiral and why did foods actually all taste the same? I then started to research and educate myself, which, with the benefit of hindsight, I should have done years ago. In the previous chapter, I mentioned how we had eaten very healthily and it slowly dawned on me how today's food has taken on a completely different dimension from that of my childhood. This led me to take a closer look at both farming methods, as discussed in the previous chapter, and the food industry.

I don't intend to give you a blow-by-blow account of the food industry's darkest secrets. If you need more in-depth knowledge on the subject, I highly recommend an excellent book by Joanna Blythman, *Swallow This: Serving up the Food Industry's Darkest Secrets*.

As discussed in the previous chapter on farming, there is a vast difference in taste between naturally produced foods and processed food. Here's the clue: one is natural and the other is not, i.e. it's manufactured in a factory. There are differences between the two. Firstly, the quality of the ingredients and, secondly, the addition of chemical additives which are added to manufactured foods to enhance flavour and preserve the foods.

Industrial food production is usually carried out in inconspicuous buildings probably located on an industrial estate far from residential areas and prying eyes. All a far cry from the tantalising appeal of the butcher, fishmonger, and fruit and veg shops mentioned in previous chapters where you were able to handpick your purchases.

Why don't we take one processed product and look carefully at the ingredients contained therein vs how the same food would be freshly prepared. Let's take the example of beef ragout.

I'd like you to paint a picture in your mind's eye of that dish (or another of your favourites) and think of its ingredients and ultimate taste. You are in your own lovely kitchen, and you've got some garlic and onions that you are going to chop and brown in some healthy olive oil. You'll brown the meat as well and then add some fresh tomatoes, red wine, beef broth, several herbs and salt and pepper, then cook the dish to perfection. Go on, I know you already have that vision in your mind and you may already be salivating at the thought! Is that how you envisage processed foods to be prepared? Well, think again. Clever marketing creates that image but the reality is far from the truth.

Normally, in fresh food preparation, the list of ingredients is comparatively short. Not so if we have to prepare for long shelf life. Another point worth noting is the quality of the ingredients. We highly recommend healthy olive oil and coconut oil to name but two, but one of the principal ingredients in food processing is vegetable oils (very high in inflammatory omega-6). This is just one example of a product which is used because it is much cheaper to buy.

Freshly prepared meals will always have a slight variation in taste which can be attributed to the source of the fresh produce used on the day, how the chef feels, whether the sun is shining, etc. However, have you ever thought why convenience food tastes nothing like a meal cooked from scratch? I certainly did! Well, there are several reasons:

- Freshly prepared ingredients can taste different especially if, one day, the cook has thrown in homemade stock or a few splashes of wine. And then there can just be the variance of the day – off or on!
- Processed food tastes the same time after time – no variance, just the same every single time. The problem is that it can be the same taste and flavour as another dish due to its everlasting ingredients. The same taste 365 days a year is the manufacturer's aim. Consistency of taste is the name of their game. Food manufacturers purchase pre-prepared ingredients, from worldwide sources, usually brought in frozen, which are then added to recipes in industrial-sized vats. The principal reason for purchasing frozen ingredients is they arrive at the factory, can be stored on site and used as required. As a result, the ingredients may not be fresh but possibly months old, albeit frozen. So, it is entirely possible that your 'made in the UK/wherever you live' could, in fact, have been imported from, say, Thailand. And these are more often than not from factory-farmed sources as well.

The only food plant where I gained first-hand knowledge was a biscuit factory when I had a summer job when I was a student, packing biscuits into packets for various retailers. There were separate runs for different brands but, to me, the biscuits looked exactly the same with the only difference to the naked eye being the packaging! I imagine it is the same principle for the production of other processed dishes whether they be meat, fish or eggs.

Turning to food flavouring – when we cook from scratch for a savoury dish, we usually add herbs and spices for flavouring. By comparison, processed food has a countless list of ingredients. Have a look at the ingredients list on any packet of crisps/chips, ready meals or yoghurts when you shop. You will be amazed and horrified at the same time. Flavourings are usually listed fairly far down the ingredients' lists. The question to ask oneself is why are supplemental factory flavourings required? Regrettably, the answer is found in the fact that processed food loses its flavour and taste and requires enhancement. Therefore, the foods require flavouring supplementation. Again, we ask: Why? Well, processed food is cooked at extremely high temperatures which can harm the ingredients thus damaging their flavour and ultimate taste.

I like to write about personal experiences to give a description. We were in South Africa recently and loved our trip. The food was great and we were able to regularly order coffee with pouring cream. Just delicious and so healthy. We were on our way to a restaurant for lunch in Muisbosskerm on the West Coast and stopped to have a coffee along the way. We ordered two coffees plus cream and waited in high expectation. When the coffees arrived, they were beautifully decorated with cream which had been whipped to an artistic state of frenzy – it was a work of art. We were in a state of high great-taste expectation. On the first sip, however, the disappointment was palpable. They had used a synthetic cream full of additives – totally unlike the taste of full-fat dairy. We moved on rapidly.

Have you ever heard the terms 'bliss point' and 'mouth feel'? I had not. Well, the definition of 'bliss point' is the amount of ingredients such as salt, sugar or fat which optimises deliciousness. Pioneering work on the 'bliss point' was carried out by an American market researcher and psychophysicist, Howard Moskowitz, known for his successful work in product creation and optimisation for foods.

The 'bliss point' is the range within which we perceive that there is neither too much nor too little but just the right amount of saltiness, sweetness or richness. Basically, our bodies favour foods that deliver these tastes and, guess what? The brain tells us that we are rewarded and makes us want to do it again, i.e. we become addicted.

In his book, *Salt Sugar Fat: How the Food Giants Hooked Us*, Michael Moss said during a presentation at Obesity Week 2018: 'This is an industry driving to get us to not just like their products but to want more and more.'

Have you ever felt like that? I know I did when I still ate processed food. I could happily eat a packet of crisps/chips and have another one an hour later and another an hour after that! For you, it may be cakes or cookies. Little did I realise that I had a craving and was actually addicted to the taste. I justified it in my mind by saying it wasn't that much – although looking back now, I realise it was.

A prime culprit ingredient is sugar. I challenge you to go to your local grocery store or supermarket and take a walk down the aisles to see the sugar content in most of the foods, sodas, bread, cereals, flavoured yoghurts – and that's before you get to the confectionery aisle! It's sugar, sugar everywhere. It's well worth the time to educate yourself on this as there is a global epidemic of 'sugarholics', which has led to the current global health figures for lifestyle diseases.

How can we have fallen hook, line and sinker for this information when, even in 1917, Rebecca Oppenheimer wrote in her book, *Diabetic Cookery*, that sugars are foods that have to be strictly forbidden and that carb sources may be used only with the doctor's permission? Remember this was before insulin was discovered in the 1920s.

Natural full-fat plain yoghurt is extremely healthy, a good source of protein and high in vitamins B and D. This is definitely a product that everybody should add to their diet. However, this is not the product that populates over 90 per cent of supermarket shelves. There you find masses of different flavourings and low-fat versions.

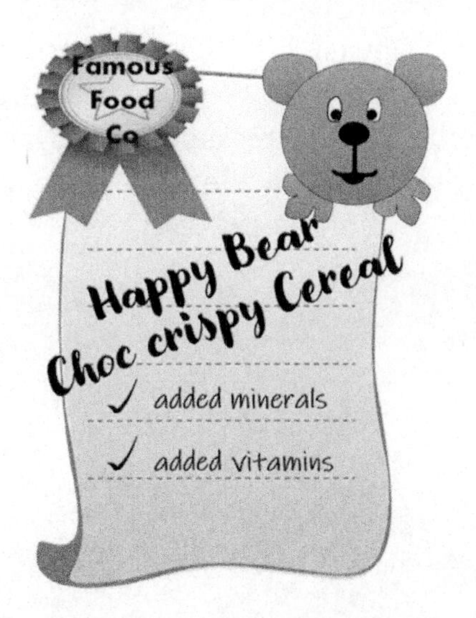

Figure 32. Fake food advertising.

The food industry often uses cute animal images to promote addictive sugar-packed products by drawing attention to other constituents such as added minerals and vitamins.

The NHS recommends choosing lower-fat or reduced-fat dairy products or even non-dairy products. This is so far removed from what we should be eating, as described in the earlier chapters of this book. Fat is not the problem. Eating fat does not make you fat.

Fat is not the problem. Eating Fat *doesn't* make you Fat!

However, this is not the advice of the NHS: 'For older children and adults, eating too much fat can contribute to excess energy intakes, leading to becoming overweight.' In addition, they recommend products with 1 per cent fat or skimmed milk! A complete contradiction to what I ate as a child, for sure, and what is healthy for us.

This advice is also followed by Diabetes UK, which provides the nutritional value of Muller Light Yoghurt on its website: each 175g serving has 13.7 carbs, i.e. four teaspoons of sugar. How can that be healthy? Oh, and did I mention the sweetener, aspartame, is also added?

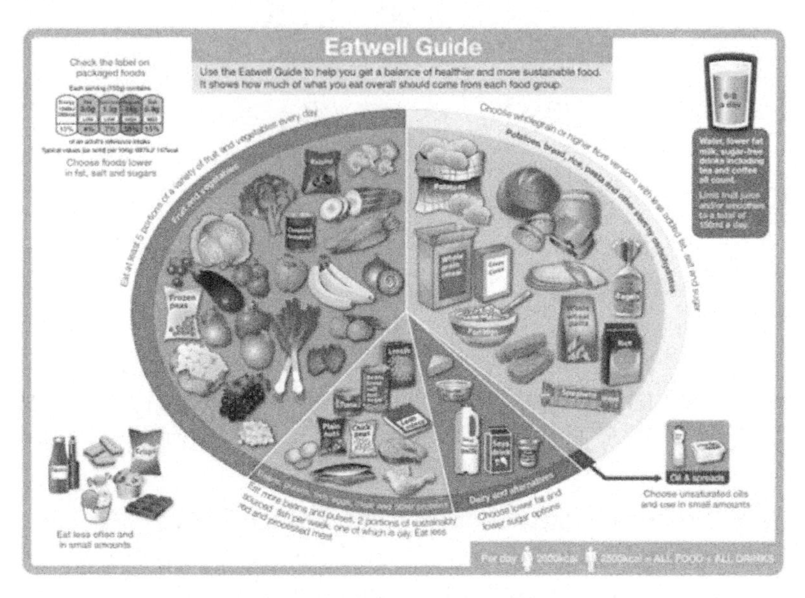

Figure 33. The UK Eatwell Guide.

Source: Public Health England in association with the Welsh Government, Food Standards Scotland and the Food Standards Agency in Northern Ireland.

The NHS also recommends that low-fat spreads can be used instead of butter! All of these guidelines are taken from the UK Eatwell Guide which pictorially recommends 'lower-fat spread, low-fat cheese, soft cheese, semi-skimmed milk and low-fat yoghurt'.

> The Health Care and Food Industries are confusing **FATS** with **CARBS.**
> *They are vilifying FATS instead of CARBS.*

Industrial Farming

Starting with crops such as wheat, barley and vegetables, let's look at the use of pesticides today. Only this morning, when we were walking the dog, we met the retired local doctor who lives nearby. We exchanged pleasantries about the weather, the crops and the subject of pesticides came up. He asked us if we remembered a time about four years ago when there was a black fly infestation of the wheat crop. We have only moved to the area recently, so we asked him to tell us. He explained that the local farmer sprayed the crop and the black flies dropped like the proverbial fly but what was more interesting was that the crop subsequently turned orange. Remember, this wheat crop formed part of the food chain!

I wrote before about the happy hens of my childhood. The reality now is far removed from that scene. Factory farming for egg-laying hens permits(!) the hens to be kept in a cage the size of an A4 sheet of paper, with a little bit of extra space for scratching and nesting. Imagine living in that confined space. It doesn't bear thinking about. Remember half the eggs eaten in the UK are laid by caged birds. High intensity of production leads to several problems, not least of which is stress. Birds, therefore, have their beaks clipped to prevent them from pecking each other (or themselves) due to stress and boredom. Animals that live in close proximity to one another, i.e. these hens, are routinely mass-medicated with antibiotics. This can lead to antibiotic resistance in humans.

Factory-farmed chickens bred for meat production fare little better. The UK's Royal Society for the Prevention of Cruelty to Animals (RSPCA) states that most meat chickens are reared in large buildings with artificial lighting with food and water strictly controlled. Low lighting encourages the birds to eat more (whilst eating weight-inducing high carb grain feed) and move around less, thereby maximising their growth rate. Five to six weeks is the normal time for the birds to reach the desired weight (2.2kg)! Due to the fast-growing methods used by breeders, the birds frequently have broken bones and suffer from lameness due to excessive weight on unformed limbs. Typically, there are at least 25,000 birds in the building and chickens are packed in together – nineteen 2kg chickens per square metre. Imagine living in that confinement – it's just horrific!

Not all birds are raised in this way, and some improvements have been made which provide for natural daylight, reduced stocking densities and straw bales for them to peck at. The luckiest ones are, however, reared free-range and organic – happy hens back in their preferred environment, nature.

Let's turn now to fish farming – this, alongside poultry, is one of the most intensive methods of all our food chain. We happily buy delicious Atlantic salmon – often blissfully unaware that these are fish farmed, packed together in their thousands. Nothing like the life of a wild salmon. I appreciate that wild salmon may not always be available and farmed may be the only option. However, these are the aspects you should consider here:

- Farmed fish are often fed on a diet of corn, soy and vegetable oil which all have higher levels of omega-6 whereas wild salmon get their omega-3 from marine lipids. Inflammation caused by excess omega-6 levels contributes to lifestyle diseases: diabetes, arthritis, heart disease, cancer and dementia. Omega-3, by comparison, is anti-inflammatory and is highly recommended.
- Overcrowding at fish farms means that fish are routinely treated with antibiotics to help prevent infection. Eating farmed salmon can, therefore, lead to antibiotic resistance in humans.
- There is also the thorny question of pesticides used in fish farming to control, for example, sea lice. Only this week, as I am writing this, there has been a disclosure that 22 tonnes of formaldehyde, which causes cancer, have been poured into cages to disinfect salmon. This has, in turn, polluted ten Scottish lochs.

Let's look now at dairy farming in the 2020s. A far cry indeed from my childhood memories. There are no available figures for the number of intensive dairy farms in the UK, but there is no doubt that both intensive farming numbers and herd size have increased dramatically since my childhood.

I feel that, regrettably, scenes of cows grazing in the fields could well become a scene from the past. Dairy farmers are under intense pressure to use factory farming methods, particularly when the value of milk is at an all-time low. This will undoubtedly lead to cows being kept indoors all year round which does have health risks for them: udder infections and lameness being two. Plus, they are being fed to produce unnaturally high amounts of milk. In the 1960s, our dairy cow, Betsy, ate grass in the field, came into the cow byre to be milked, and then went back out again into the field to eat grass again. The only supplementary feed she had was hay in winter.

You may have seen TV programmes showing cows whose udders are so distended they can hardly walk; in fact, it's more like a duck waddling. It is also important to understand that cows are herd animals who love being outside in nature and, whilst they love each other's company, if they are kept housed in close proximity to one another, have a tendency to become anxious and also aggressive. A bit like humans who are kept together against their will!

US-style mega farms are now prevalent in the UK and number over 800. This figure is dwarfed by the large-scale farming numbers from the US, which has 50,000 facilities classified as concentrated animal feeding operations (CAFOs) and a further quarter of a million industrial-scale facilities. In the last six years alone, in the UK there has been a 26 per cent rise in intensive factory farming. The most prominent numbers are for poultry and pigs.

Concerns from critics include local residents who are concerned about odour and noise from these mega farms, as well as concerns in general regarding animal welfare and disease outbreaks. Of great concern is the fact that animals are never allowed to be in their natural habitat. Anyone who knows animals will know that they just love the freedom of being outside in their herd eating fresh pasture.

Poultry farms tend to have the largest numbers – in some cases, over 1 million per facility. Pigs come a distant second in numbers with about 23,000 pigs, and the largest intensive beef cattle farm has around 3,000, although there are currently proposals to increase the numbers.

It is important to remember that factory farming is driven by profit. This approach has little concern for animal welfare and is totally designed to maximise production whilst minimising costs.

Research from the Bureau of Investigate Journalism and the Guardian reveals, in an article in early June 2020, industrial-scale beef fattening units with herds of up to 3,000 cattle have now been established in the UK. Cattle are held in grassless pens for extended periods rather than grazing or being raised in barns. These animals have little or no access to nature. A far cry from previous days.

Industrial-scale proponents say it enables farmers to raise the cattle efficiently and profitably but critics are concerned that there are welfare issues.

Could these smaller units, in comparison to America's huge units, be just the thin end of the wedge? Will the US-style mega beef farm be replicated in the UK? Well, as mentioned above, it is happening already. The relentless push for more product for less money could well drive this. We, however, definitely advocate quality over quantity every time.

Sitting on the arm of an armchair, when I was a kid, pretending I was a cowboy on a horse charging over the prairies of the Wild West, I watched cowboys lassoing cattle under endless blue skies – such a romantic picture in my tomboy mind. And there was not a mega farm in sight! Changed days indeed!

Who is driving this trend for food produced in this way? And who are the principal buyers from these mega farms? The supermarkets and fast food operators of course!

Now, I don't mean to infer that all farmers use these intensive methods. That is not the case and, in fact, in recent years there has been a welcome trend to revert to successful methods used in the past. These include self-manured pastures for their animals, allowing them to live in their natural herds, and keeping their farms pesticide-free thereby allowing a variety of plants to grow and allowing animals to self-select their nutrition. So, it can be done, and we certainly endorse their efforts.

Are We on the Brink of a Worldwide Revolution on How we Buy Food?

Let's hope so!

As the worldwide COVID-19 pandemic takes hold, we should be asking ourselves questions like 'Where is our food coming from?', 'What is the traceability of this product?' and 'Should we be concentrating on quality rather than quantity?'

We are definitely seeing a greater awareness regarding food sources. It is, perhaps, timely to mention a recent infographic published by Oxfam America showing how just ten multi-billion-dollar food and drink companies control 70 per cent of what we eat today. Yes, 70 per cent of what we eat! Interesting – and scary at the same time.

These companies all produce processed foods, the health effects of which are fully discussed in Part 1 of the book. So, let's reflect on our eating habits and, taking account of the information you have now gleaned from this book, make just one adjustment – take that first step towards eating more healthily sourced nutritious produce.

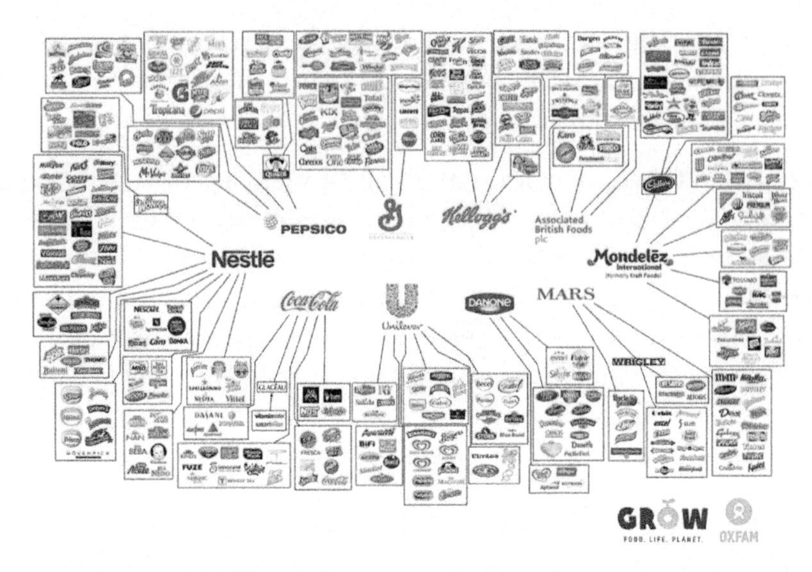

Figure 34. Ten multi-billion-dollar companies control 70 per cent of processed food and drink production.

Farm shops and ethical producers have had to reinvent themselves during this pandemic by finding new avenues to sell their fresh produce. Whilst some opportunities have dried up due to the closure of the hospitality industry, other avenues have opened. These include an upsurge in demand for home deliveries. With no farmers' markets available during the pandemic, we have greatly benefited from home delivery both for grass-fed meats and organic leafy vegetables from local suppliers. The service has been prompt, friendly and delivered with a smile, and we have really enjoyed the experience.

There has definitely been a rise in local home delivery schemes, with some producers linking together to provide a one-stop online shop. These producers can, therefore, provide direct sales to their local market through doorstep deliveries.

Will consumers have developed a real love for the taste of these products and will this continue when normal shopping patterns resume? Will we remain loyal to our local suppliers rather than return to the bland offerings of the supermarkets? Time will tell, but we very much hope so. It will benefit both the local supplier and, more importantly, the health of the consumer.

Liz Bowles, Associate Director for Farming and Land Use at the Soil Association UK, says, 'There is a huge opportunity to think about what food looks like, not only the cost of it, but what goes into it, how it's produced and what impact it is having on our climate, the health of our consumers and nature. I think a lot of people are feeling more connected to food and are really thinking about where it comes from,' adding, 'perhaps a shorter supply chain is better.'

As previously mentioned, there has been an upsurge in local food supplier box deliveries direct to households, resulting in a much shorter food supply chain. In the instance of delicious grass-fed beef, the local farmer actually sells direct to his customer and the same method applies to the local fruit and veg supplier. Or the suppliers can link together and agree that one of them does the delivery, with a central delivery point to their distribution service. So, there is a maximum of two to three stages in the 'farm fresh' process.

Are we willing to pay a little more for locally produced food rather than just buy everything from the local supermarket? We think a lot of people would be willing to do so, particularly bearing in mind that we find that quality beats quantity every time.

We hope that the changes we have seen short term will be followed through to a long-term food revolution. Ultimately, this will have enormous health benefits for us all. Will you be part of it?

Important Points:

- Focus on seeking out quality food rather than quantity.
- Champion ethically produced food from local suppliers.

Chapter 8

PRACTICAL TIPS – WHAT TO DO

'He who has health has hope, and he who has hope has everything.'

Arabian Proverb

You will have gleaned from previous chapters that, for decades, we have been fed (forgive the pun) the wrong advice that has dramatically increased lifestyle diseases including obesity, type 2 diabetes, heart disease and dementia. Regrettably, you may be suffering from one or more of these diseases yourself and now realise that the question you should have been asking is, 'What if education has been wrong all along, and the information that we have been taught based on the dietary guidelines is totally incorrect?' With your new-found knowledge, you will realise that in the past you didn't know what you didn't know, whereas now you understand that, in fact, you know what you didn't know previously! Now there is a need for a fresh roadmap to health for yourself. So, what are you going to do with this fresh knowledge and where is the roadmap?

Knowledge is King

Be assured, none of this is your fault. We all do what we can with the knowledge we are taught and believe to be correct. We know we did.

Let's start with an example first to demonstrate the issue.

This example is taken from the NHS Nutrition and Dietetic Service in England, whose guidance comes from the UK *Eatwell Guide* or the similar *Food Pyramid* in the US. Their website proudly states that they are giving some ideas for healthy eating advice. We have taken a snapshot of their 24-hr suggested meals from their leaflet and calculated the net carb values.

Meal	Food	Net Carbs(g)
Breakfast	100g Oats porridge *plus* 125mL semi-skimmed milk	63g
Lunch	Sandwich: 2 slices whole wheat bread + ham, lettuce & tomato	31g
Snack	Packet of crisps *or* 2 biscuits	15g
Dinner	128g Spaghetti *plus* 113g Bolognaise sauce *plus* Salad	43g
Total Net Carbs		**152g**

Figure 35. Meal guidance from NHS Nutrition and Dietetic Service, Leicestershire.

A total of 152g of net carbs – the equivalent of 38 teaspoons of sugar! The UK NHS guidelines for sugar intake are 30g of *free sugars* per adult – these guidelines take *no account of the sugar content of bread, pasta, grains, etc.*, which is the whole problem. The guidelines are, in fact, promoting the development of type 2 diabetes (and other diseases), and for patients already diagnosed with diabetes, ensuring that they will never get better, but become ever more dependent on medication with their disease pursuing a relentlessly progressive course.

It brings us back to the very basics of nutrition. Not knowing the macronutrient composition of the food that you eat and, on top of that, not understanding that the breakdown product of sugar and starch is the same, in other words, glucose, then you cannot possibly understand what a healthy eating programme is.

Basic Nutrition Lesson
Sugar breaks down to *glucose*
Starch breaks down to *glucose*

It's not that difficult, is it?

It brings to mind the quote from the *Postgrad Med J* blog referring to one of the first things that new medical students are told early on: '50% of what we teach you over the next five years will be wrong, or inaccurate. Sadly, we don't know which 50%.' The really disturbing part is that, with regard to nutrition, the science is there, but the teachers have forgotten it.

Thus, we see that the guidelines are misleading, to say the least. What is so frustrating is that the knowledge was already known and documented in Rebecca Oppenheimer's previously mentioned book, *Diabetic Cookery Recipes and Menus*, published a century ago in 1917. Her advice was to eat butter, cream cheeses, meat, poultry, fish and eggs and to completely avoid sugar, bread, flour, grains, sweet fruits and dried fruits. Here was the wisdom of the past and so sadly lost in time.

You will recollect that, in the first chapter of this book, we asked the question 'Is it about the quantity (of the food that we eat) or about the quality?' This question boils down to 'Is it the calorific content or is it the type of foodstuffs we consume?'. You will now understand that the answer is very definitely the latter. Knowing what foods to eat, and then consuming them, will definitely lead you to a healthier life free from lifestyle diseases.

Okay, so What to Do?

All the information so far highlights the health problems associated with a high carbohydrate diet. It stands to reason, then, that cutting your daily carbohydrate intake and making up the loss with extra good fat and protein is the way to go. When you do this consistently, you will experience one or many of the following:

- Reduced sugar addiction
- Improved overall health
- Weight loss
- Enhanced mental focus (less brain fog)
- Improved mood
- Improved physical performance
- Few (if any) food cravings
- Better sleep
- Improved blood glucose levels (lower levels)
- No hunger pangs
- More energy
- Improved blood pressure (lower blood pressure)

Doesn't that sound good? Just think what a difference that would make to your life. Now, to achieve that, these are the guidelines that you need to follow – we are sure that Rebecca Oppenheimer would approve.

Healthy Eating Guidelines

- Avoid all processed foods: pre-packed, pre-boxed and fast food.
- Exclude sugar (in all its forms) and fructose (*added* or *natural* in fruit with high fructose content).
- Eliminate all grains (including gluten free alternatives).
- Eliminate all refined carbs (anything made from white or whole meal flour).
- Eat carbohydrates from green leafy vegetables and berries.
- Eat ample amounts of good fats (always full-fat products) e.g.
  meat, butter, fish, eggs, cheese, coconut oil, nuts, avocado.

Figure 36. Healthy eating guidelines.

Now you are thinking, how on earth am I going to do that? What is left for me to eat?! If you are like us, that was a question we were asking ourselves. There is a lot of information out there on the internet, some good and some bad. If you are not sure how to channel the advice into your own meal plans or menus, then you should find a programme that will help you. Now you are asking yourself: *What should the correct programme consist of?*

We recommend a programme that is evidence based and backed by science. It needs to be a real-food programme, not one based on shakes and juices (high in sugar anyway) for a quick fix, with simple, tasty real-food menus that will give you a solid platform for a healthy way of life. Happy hunting!

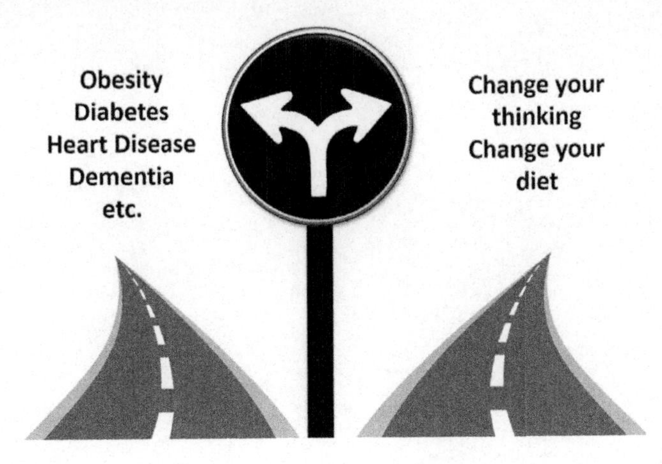

End Notes

We hope that after reading this book you will feel as passionately as we do that the correct information must be shared with everybody so that people can make informed decisions about their own lives and health. We owe it to everybody. How long are we going to be held hostage by the food and drink industry that is turning out a huge variety of highly refined processed foods, drinks laden with glucose and unhealthy cheap vegetable oils? It is time that we, the public, start voicing our concerns and give a clear message: enough is enough!

The medical profession has a lot to explain. The key issue here is a lack of knowledge. Nutrition must be taught as a serious subject in medical school – the real science and not the standard misinformation-sponsored-research from food, drink and pharmaceutical industries. Doctors must be made aware that they are being exploited by the big food and drug companies.

And, last but not least, why not give a copy of this book to your GP the next time you go for your consultation, especially if they advise you to follow the national nutrition guidelines or want to prescribe you a statin to bring your cholesterol levels down?

The End

Or is it a new beginning for you?

Chapter 9

REFERENCES

Introduction

Healthcare Media, 2020, *Top Chronic Diseases Behind Payer Spending and How to Prevent Them*. https://healthpayerintelligence.com/news/top-chronic-diseases-behind-payer-spending-and-how-to-prevent-them

Chapter 1: The Basics of Food

Berger ME, Smesny S, Kim SW, et al. Omega-6 to omega-3 polyunsaturated fatty acid ratio and subsequent mood disorders in young people with at-risk mental states: a 7-year longitudinal study. *Transl Psychiatry*. 2017;7(8):e1220. doi:10.1038/tp.2017.190

Blasbalg TL, Hibbeln JR, Ramsden CE, Majchrzak SF, Rawlings RR. Changes in consumption of omega-3 and omega-6 fatty acids in the United States during the 20th century. *Am J Clin Nutr*. 2011;93(5):950-962. doi:10.3945/ajcn.110.006643

Committees on Toxicity (COT). *Annual Report* 2013. https://cot.food.gov.uk/sites/default/files/Annual%20Report%202013%20for%20web_0.pdf

Committees on Toxicity (COT). *Annual Report* 2015. https://cot.food.gov.uk/sites/default/files/annualreport2015.pdf

Deol P, Evans JR, Dhahbi J, et al. Soybean oil is more obesogenic and diabetogenic than coconut oil and fructose in mouse: Potential role for the liver. *PLoS One*. 2015;10(7):e0132672. doi:10.1371/journal.pone.0132672

Deol P, Kozlova E, Valdez M, et al. Dysregulation of hypothalamic gene expression and the oxytocinergic system by soybean oil diets in male mice. *Endocrinology*. 2020;161(2):bqz044. doi:10.1210/endocr/bqz044

Dyall SC. Long-chain omega-3 fatty acids and the brain: a review of the independent and shared effects of EPA, DPA and DHA. *Front Aging Neurosci*. 2015;7:52. doi:10.3389/fnagi.2015.00052

Ede G, *Your Brain on Plants: Micronutrients and Mental Health.* https://www.diagnosisdiet.com/full-article/micronutrients-and-mental-health

Harcombe Z. *The Obesity Epidemic*. UK: Columbus Publishing Ltd; 2015.

Keith L. *The Vegetarian Myth*. CA: Flashpoint Press; 2009.

Masterjohn C, *The Ultimate Vitamin K2 Resource*. https://chrismasterjohnphd.com/blog/2016/12/09/the-ultimate-vitamin-k2-resource

McNamara RK, Carlson SE. Role of omega-3 fatty acids in brain development and function: potential implications for the pathogenesis and prevention of psychopathology. *Prostaglandins Leukot Essent Fatty Acids*. 2006;75(4-5):329-349. doi:10.1016/j.plefa.2006.07.010

Tripkovic L, Lambert H, Hart K, et al. Comparison of vitamin D2 and vitamin D3 supplementation in raising serum 25-hydroxyvitamin D status: A systematic review and meta-analysis. *Am J Clin Nutr*. 2012;95(6):1357-1364. doi:10.3945/ajcn.111.031070 van Vliet S, Burd NA, van Loon LJ. The skeletal muscle anabolic response to plant- versus animal-based protein consumption. *J Nutr.* 2015;145(9):1981-1991. doi:10.3945/jn.114.204305

Zhong L, Goldberg MS, Parent ME, Hanley JA. Risk of developing lung cancer in relation to exposure to fumes from Chinese-style cooking. *Scand J Work Environ Health*. 1999;25(4):309-316. doi:10.5271/sjweh.440

Zhong L, Goldberg MS, Gao YT, Jin F. Lung cancer and indoor air pollution arising from Chinese-style cooking among nonsmoking women living in Shanghai, China. *Epidemiology*. 1999;10(5):488-494.

Zhao Y, Wang S, Aunan K, Seip HM, Hao J. Air pollution and lung cancer risks in China – a meta-analysis. *Sci Total Environ*. 2006;366(2-3):500-513. doi:10.1016/j.scitotenv.2005.10.010

Chapter 2: What did our Ancestors Eat?

NHS. 2019. *The Eatwell Guide*. https://www.nhs.uk/live-well/eat-well/the-eatwell-guide/

Noakes R, Proudfoot J, Creed S-A. *The Real Meal Revolution*. London, UK: Robinson; 2015.

Stefansson V. Adventures in Diet. *Harper's Monthly Magazine*. 1935. Internet Archive Copy. https://archive.org/stream/adventuresindiet00stef_0/adventuresindiet00stef_0_djvu.txt

Taubes G. *Why We Get Fat*, New York, NY: Alfred A. Knopf; 2011.

Teicholz N. *The Big Fat Surprise*. New York, NY: Simon and Schuster; 2014.

Chapter 3: The War between Fat and Sugar

Agha M, Agha R. The rising prevalence of obesity: Part A: Impact on public health. *Int J Surg Oncol* (N Y). 2017;2(7):e17. doi:10.1097/IJ9.0000000000000017

Anderson KM, Castelli WP, Levy D. Cholesterol and mortality. 30 years of follow-up from the Framingham study. *JAMA*. 1987;257(16):2176-2180. doi:10.1001/jama.257.16.2176

Blasbalg TL, Hibbeln JR, Ramsden CE, Majchrzak SF, Rawlings RR. Changes in consumption of omega-3 and omega-6 fatty acids in the United States during the 20th century. *Am J Clin Nutr*. 2011;93(5):950-962. doi:10.3945/ajcn.110.006643

Campbell GD. Diabetes in Asians and Africans in and around Durban. *S Afr Med J*. 1963;37:1195-1208.

CDC. Trends in intake of energy and macronutrients – United States, 1971-2000. *MMWR Morb Mortal Wkly Rep*. 2004;53(4):80-82.

CDC, *Estimated Hypertension Prevalence, Treatment, and Control Among U.S. Adults*, 2020. https://millionhearts.hhs.gov/data-reports/hypertension-prevalence.html#Figure1

CDC. *National Diabetes Statistics Report*, 2020. https://www.cdc.gov/diabetes/data/statistics/statistics-report.html

Cleave TL. *The Saccharine Disease*. Bristol, UK: John Wright & Sons Ltd, Stonebridge Press; 1974

Gale EAM. The rise of childhood type 1 diabetes in the 20th century. *Diabetes*, 2002; 51:3353-3361

Guardian The, 2016, *The sugar conspiracy*. https://www.theguardian.com/society/2016/apr/07/the-sugar-conspiracy-robert-lustig-john-yudkin

Gross LS, Li L, Ford ES, Liu S. Increased consumption of refined carbohydrates and the epidemic of type 2 diabetes in the United States: An ecologic assessment. *Am J Clin Nutr*. 2004;79(5):774-779. doi:10.1093/ajcn/79.5.774

Hales CM, Carroll MD, Fryar CD, Ogden CL. Prevalence of Obesity and Severe Obesity Among Adults: United States, 2017-2018. *NCHS Data Brief*. 2020;(360):1-8.

Hallfrisch J. Metabolic effects of dietary fructose. *FASEB J*. 1990;4(9):2652-2660. doi:10.1096/fasebj.4.9.2189777

Harcombe Z, 2010, *Cholesterol & heart disease – there is a relationship, but it's not what you think.* https://www.zoeharcombe.com/2010/11/cholesterol-heart-disease-there-is-a-relationship-but-its-not-what-you-think/

Harcombe Z, Baker JS, DiNicolantonio JJ, Grace F, Davies B. Evidence from randomised controlled trials does not support current dietary fat guidelines: a systematic review and meta-analysis. *Open Heart*. 2016;3(2):e000409. Published 2016 Aug 8. doi:10.1136/openhrt-2016-000409

Harcombe Z, Baker JS, Davies B. Evidence from prospective cohort studies does not support current dietary fat guidelines: a systematic review and meta-analysis. *Br J Sports Med*. 2017;51(24):1743-1749. doi:10.1136/bjsports-2016-096550

Heidemann C, Scheidt-Nave C. Prevalence, incidence and mortality of diabetes mellitus in adults in Germany – A review in the framework of the Diabetes Surveillance. *Journal of Health Monitoring* 2017 2(3) DOI 10.17886/RKI-GBE-2017-062 Robert Koch Institute, Berlin.

Johnson RJ, Segal MS, Sautin Y, et al. Potential role of sugar (fructose) in the epidemic of hypertension, obesity and the metabolic syndrome, diabetes, kidney disease, and cardiovascular disease. *Am J Clin Nutr*. 2007;86(4):899-906. doi:10.1093/ajcn/86.4.899

Kearns CE, Schmidt LA, Glantz SA. (2016). Sugar industry and coronary heart disease research: A historical analysis of internal industry documents. *JAMA Internal Medicine*, 2016;176(11):1680-1685. https://doi.org/10.1001/jamainternmed.2016.5394

Kendrick M. *The Great Cholesterol Con*: The Truth About What Really Causes Heart Disease and How to Avoid It. London, UK: John Blake; 2007.

Kendrick M. *A Statin Nation*. London, UK: John Blake; 2018.

Keys A. Normal plasma cholesterol in a man who eats 25 eggs a day. *NEJM*. 1991;325(8):584. doi:10.1056/NEJM199108223250814

Malhotra A, O'Neill D. *The Pioppi Diet*. UK: Penguin Books; 2017.

Mann GV. Diet-Heart: End of an era. *NEJM*. 1977;297(12):644-650. doi:10.1056/ NEJM197709222971206

Mann GV. The clinical trials. In: Mann GV, Ed. *Coronary Heart Disease. The Dietary Sense and Nonsense. An Evaluation by Scientists*. London, UK: Janus Publishing Company; 1993:61-75.

McGandy RB, et al., Dietary fats, carbohydrates and atherosclerotic vascular disease. *NEJM*. 1967. PMID: 5339699 Review.

New York Times. 2015. *Coca-Cola Funds Scientists Who Shift Blame for Obesity Away from Bad Diets*. https://well.blogs.nytimes.com/2015/08/09/coca-cola-funds-scientists-who-shift-blame-for-obesity-away-from-bad-diets/

New York Times. 2016. *How the Sugar Industry Shifted Blame to Fat*. https://www.nytimes.com/2016/09/13/well/eat/how-the-sugar-industry-shifted-blame-to-fat.html

Noakes T. 2019. *CrossFit: It's the Insulin Resistance, Stupid: Part 9.* https://www.crossfit.com/essentials/its-the-insulin-resistance-stupid-part-9

Noakes T. 2020. *CrossFit: Ancel Keys' Cholesterol Con, Part 1 & Part 2*. https://www.crossfit.com/health/ancel-keys-cholesterol-con-part-1

Ramsden CE, Zamora D, Majchrzak-Hong S, Faurot KR, Broste SK, Frantz RP, Davis JM, Ringel A, Suchindran CM, Hibbeln JR. Re-evaluation of the traditional diet-heart hypothesis: Analysis of Recovered data from Minnesota Coronary Experiment (1968-73). *BMJ (Online)*. 2016; 353. https://doi.org/10.1136/bmj.i1246

Taubes G. Nutrition. The soft science of dietary fat. *Science*. 2001;291(5513):2536-2545. doi:10.1126/science.291.5513.2536

Taubes G. *Good Calories, Bad Calories: Fats, Carbs, and the Controversial Science of Diet and Health*, New York, NY: Anchor Books; 2008.

Taubes G. *The Case Against Sugar*, London, UK: Portobello Books; 2018.

Teicholz N. *The Big Fat Surprise*. New York, NY: Simon and Schuster; 2014.

Time Magazine, 1961, *Medicine: The Fat of the Land.* http://content.time.com/time/subscriber/article/0,33009,828721-1,00.html

US Department of Health and Human Services and Department of Agriculture. *Nutrition and Your Health: Dietary Guidelines for Americans*. Washington, DC: US Government Printing Office; 1980.

Ward ZJ, Bleich SN, Cradock AL, et al. Projected U.S. state-level prevalence of adult obesity and severe obesity. *NEJM*. 2019;381(25):2440-2450. doi:10.1056/NEJMsa1909301

Yerushalmy J, Hilleboe HE. Fat in the diet and mortality from heart disease. A Methodological note. *New Y State J Med*.1957;57: 2343-2354.

Yudkin J. Camb MRCP. Diet and Coronary Thrombosis Hypothesis and Fact. *Lancet*. 1957;270:155-162.

Yudkin J. The Low-Carbohydrate Diet in the Treatment of Obesity, *Postgraduate Medicine*, 1972;51(5):151-154, DOI: 10.1080/00325481.1972.11698244

Yudkin J. *Pure, White and Deadly*, Revised edition. England: Penguin Life; 1986.

Chapter 4: Insulin Resistance

Fox CS, Pencina MJ, Meigs JB, Vasan RS, Levitzky YS, D'Agostino RB Sr. Trends in the incidence of type 2 diabetes mellitus from the 1970s to the 1990s: The Framingham Heart Study. *Circulation*. 2006;113(25):2914-2918. doi:10.1161/CIRCULATIONAHA.106.613828

Fung J. *The Obesity Code*. London, UK: Scribe Publications; 2016.

Janson J, Laedtke T, Parisi JE, O'Brien P, Petersen RC, Butler PC. Increased risk of type 2 diabetes in Alzheimer disease. *Diabetes*. 2004;53(2):474-481. doi:10.2337/diabetes.53.2.474

Kim B, Feldman EL. Insulin resistance as a key link for the increased risk of cognitive impairment in the metabolic syndrome. *Exp Mol Med*. 2015;47(3):e149. Published 2015 Mar 13. doi:10.1038/emm.2015.3

Noakes T. 2019. *CrossFit: It's the Insulin Resistance, Stupid: Parts 1–11.* https://www.crossfit.com/essentials/its-the-insulin-resistance-stupid-part-1

Ott A, Stolk RP, van Harskamp F, Pols HA, Hofman A, Breteler MM. Diabetes mellitus and the risk of dementia: The Rotterdam Study. *Neurology*. 1999;53(9):1937-1942. doi:10.1212/wnl.53.9.1937

Volek J, Phinney S. *The Art and Science of Low Carbohydrate Living*. Great Britain: Amazon; 2011.

Chapter 5: Dietary Diseases

Diabetes and TOFI

Athinarayanan SJ, Adams RN, Hallberg SJ, et al. Long-term effects of a novel continuous remote care intervention including nutritional ketosis for the management of type 2 diabetes: A 2-year non-randomized clinical trial. *Front Endocrinol (Lausanne)*. 2019;10:348. Published 2019 Jun 5. doi:10.3389/fendo.2019.00348

Conus F, Rabasa-Lhoret R, Péronnet F. Characteristics of metabolically obese normal-weight (MONW) subjects. *Appl Physiol Nutr Metab*. 2007;32(1):4-12. doi:10.1139/h06-092

Diet Doctor. 2018. *Dr. Gary Fettke exonerated! Receives apology from Regulators.* https://www.dietdoctor.com/dr-gary-fettke-exonerated-receives-apology-from-regulators

Evert AB, Dennison M, Gardner CD, et al. Nutrition therapy for adults with diabetes or prediabetes: A consensus report. *Diabetes Care*. 2019;42(5):731-754. doi:10.2337/dci19-0014

Guardian The. 2006. *Are you a Tofi? (That's thin on the outside, fat inside)*: https://www.theguardian.com/science/2006/dec/10/medicineandhealth.health

Noakes T, Sboros M. *Lore of Nutrition*. Cape Town, South Africa: Penguin; 2017.

Ruderman NB, Schneider SH, Berchtold P. The "metabolically-obese," normal-weight individual. *Am J Clin Nutr*. 1981;34(8):1617-1621. doi:10.1093/ajcn/34.8.1617

Unwin D. *NICE Endorsed Sugar Equivalence Infographics*. https://phcuk.org/wp-content/uploads/2020/05/Common-Foods-21.05.2020.jpg

Unwin D. *Seven Years of Low-carb*, PHC Virtual Conference 2020. https://www.youtube.com/watch?v=RUH7epLxkV8

Cancer

Evans JMM, Donnelly LA, Emslie-Smith AM, Alessi DR, Morris AD. Metformin and reduced risk of cancer in diabetic patients. *British Medical Journal*. 2005;330(7503): 1304-1305. https://doi.org/10.1136/bmj.38415.708634.F7

Hagihara K, Kajimoto K, Osaga S, Naga, N, Shimosegawa E, Nakata H, Saito H, Nakano M, Takeuchi M, Kanki H, Kagitani-Shimono K, & Kijima T. Promising effect of a new ketogenic diet regimen in patients with advanced cancer. *Nutrients*. 2020;12(5):1473. https://doi.org/10.3390/nu12051473

Hsu PP, Sabatini DM. Cancer cell metabolism: Warburg and beyond. *Cell*. 2008;134(5), 703-707. https://doi.org/10.1016/j.cell.2008.08.021

Klement RJ, Kämmerer U. Is there a role for carbohydrate restriction in the treatment and prevention of cancer? *Nutr Metab (Lond)*. 2011;8:75. doi:10.1186/1743-7075-8-75

Lende TH, Austdal M, Bathen TF, Varhaugvik AE, Skaland I, Gudlaugsson E, Egeland NG, Lunde S, Akslen LA, Jonsdottir K, Janssen EAM, Søiland H, Baak JPA. Metabolic consequences of perioperative oral carbohydrates in breast cancer patients – An explorative study. *BMC Cancer*, 2019;19(1). https://doi.org/10.1186/s12885-019-6393-7

Li W, Zhang X, Sang H, Zhou Y, Shang C, Wang Y & Zhu H. Effects of hyperglycemia on the progression of tumor diseases. *Journal of Experimental and Clinical Cancer Research*, 2019;38,1. BioMed Central Ltd. https://doi.org/10.1186/s13046-019-1309-6

Seyfried TN, Flores RE, Poff AM, D'Agostino DP. Cancer as a metabolic disease: Implications for novel therapeutics. In *Carcinogenesis*, 2014; 35(3):515-527. Oxford University Press. https://doi.org/10.1093/carcin/bgt480

Seyfried TN, Yu G, Maroon JC, D'Agostino DP. Press-pulse: A novel therapeutic strategy for the metabolic management of cancer. *Nutrition and Metabolism*. 2017;14(1). https://doi.org/10.1186/s12986-017-0178-2

Seyfried TN, Mukherjee P, Iyikesici MS, Slocum A, Kalamian M, Spinosa JP, Chinopoulos, C. Consideration of ketogenic metabolic therapy as a complementary or alternative approach for managing breast cancer. *Frontiers in Nutrition*. 2020;7. Frontiers Media S.A. https://doi.org/10.3389/fnut.2020.00021

Srinivasan S, Guha M, Kashina A, Avadhani NG. Mitochondrial dysfunction and mitochondrial dynamics – The cancer connection. *Biochimica et Biophysica Acta* – Bioenergetics. 2017a;1858(8):602-614. Elsevier B.V. https://doi.org/10.1016/j.bbabio.2017.01.004

Tan-Shalaby JL, Carrick J, Edinger K, Genovese D, Liman AD, Passero VA, Shah RB. Modified Atkins diet in advanced malignancies – Final results of a safety and feasibility trial within the Veterans Affairs Pittsburgh Healthcare System. *Nutrition and Metabolism*. 2016;13(1). https://doi.org/10.1186/s12986-016-0113-y

Tan-Shalaby J, Ketogenic Diets and Cancer: Emerging Evidence. *Federal Practitioner*. 2018; Feb 24. https://www.mdedge.com/fedprac/search?search_api_views_fulltext=Tan+Shalaby

vander Heiden MG, Cantley LC, Thompson CB. Understanding the Warburg Effect: The metabolic requirements of cell proliferation. *Science*, 2009;324(5930):1029-1033. https://doi.org/10.1126/science.1160809

Dementia and Mood Disorders

de La Monte SM. Brain insulin resistance and deficiency as therapeutic targets in Alzheimer's Disease. *Current Alzheimer Research*. 2012;9.

de la Monte, SM. Insulin Resistance and neurodegeneration: Progress towards the development of new therapeutics for Alzheimer's Disease. *Drugs*. 2017;77(1):47-65. Springer International Publishing. https://doi.org/10.1007/s40265-016-0674-0

Gudala K, Bansal D, Schifano F, Bhansali A. Diabetes mellitus and risk of dementia: A meta-analysis of prospective observational studies. *J Diabetes Investig*. 2013;4(6):640-650. doi:10.1111/jdi.12087

Jacka FN, O'Neil A, Opie R, et al. A randomised controlled trial of dietary improvement for adults with major depression (the 'SMILES' trial). *BMC Med*. 2017;15(23). https://doi.org/10.1186/s12916-017-0791-y

Lamers F, Milaneschi Y, Smit JH, Schoevers RA, Wittenberg G, Penninx BWJH. Longitudinal association between depression and inflammatory markers: Results from the Netherlands study of depression and anxiety [published correction appears in Biol Psychiatry. 2020 Jun 15;87(12):1083]. *Biol Psychiatry*. 2019;85(10):829-837. doi:10.1016/j.biopsych.2018.12.020

Najjar S, Pearlman DM, Alper K, Najjar A, Devinsky O. Neuroinflammation and psychiatric illness. *J Neuroinflammation*. 2013;10:43. doi:10.1186/1742-2094-10-43

Neth BJ, Craft S. Insulin resistance and Alzheimer's disease: Bioenergetic linkages. In Frontiers in *Aging Neuroscience*. 2017;

9(OCT). Frontiers Media S.A.
https://doi.org/10.3389/fnagi.2017.00345

Other Diseases

Crofts CAP, Zinn C, Wheldon M, Schofield G. Hyperinsulinemia: A unifying theory of chronic disease? *Diabesity*. 2015;1(4):34-43. doi:10.15562/diabesity.2015.19.

Scofield G, Zinn C, Rodger C. *What the Fat?* San Francisco, CA: Weldon Owen; 2015.

Chapter 6: The Impact of Farming Methods

NFU online. *Food standards Petition*. 2020. https://www.nfuonline.com/news/latest-news/food-standards-petition/

Pesticide Action Network UK. 2018. *The Hidden Rise of UK Pesticide Use: Fact-checking an Industry Claim*. https://issuu.com/pan-uk/docs/the_hidden_rise_of_uk_pesticide_use?e=28041656/59634015

Chapter 7: Processed Foods and Industrial Farming

Blythman J. *Swallow This*. London, UK: Fourth Estate; 2015.

Bureau of Investigative Journalism. 2017. *The rise of the "megafarm": How British meat is made*. https://www.thebureauinvestigates.com/stories/2017-07-17/megafarms-uk-intensive-farming-meat

Diabetes UK. *Yogurt*. https://www.diabetes.org.uk/guide-to-diabetes/enjoy-food/eating-with-diabetes/diabetes-food-myths/yogurts

Guardian, The. 2017. *UK has nearly 800 livestock mega farms, investigation reveals.* https://www.theguardian.com/environment/2017/jul/17/uk-has-nearly-800-livestock-mega-farms-investigation-reveals

Moss M. *Salt, Sugar, Fat*. UK: WH Allen, Random House Group; 2014.

NFU Online. 2020. *Our food standards campaign: The journey so far.* https://www.nfuonline.com/back-british-farming/campaign-news/our-food-standards-campaign-the-journey-so-far/

NHS. 2019. *The Eatwell Guide.* https://www.nhs.uk/live-well/eat-well/the-eatwell-guide/

NHS. 2020. *Eating processed foods.* https://www.nhs.uk/live-well/eat-well/what-are-processed-foods/

Oppenheimer RW. 1919. *Diabetic Cookery, Recipes and Menus*, Hathi Trust Digital Library. https://babel.hathitrust.org/cgi/pt?id=wu.89042014746

RSPCA. 2020. *Farming meat chickens.* https://www.rspca.org.uk/adviceandwelfare/farm/meatchickens/farming

Chapter 8: Practical Tips – What to Do

Hillman T. 2014. Fifty percent of what you were taught is wrong... *Postgrad Med J.* https://blogs.bmj.com/pmj/2014/05/30/50-of-what-you-are-taught-is-wrong/

NHS Leicestershire Nutrition and Dietetic Service. 2017. *RECIPE AND MENU IDEAS FOR HEALTHY EATING:* https://www.lnds.nhs.uk/Library/RecipeandMenuIdeasforHealthyEatingFeb17LNDS089.pdf

REFERENCES

Oppenheimer RW. 1919. *Diabetic Cookery, Recipes and Menus*, Hathi Trust Digital Library.
https://babel.hathitrust.org/cgi/pt?id=wu.89042014746

GLOSSARY

Amino acids – the basic building blocks of protein are organic compounds composed of nitrogen, carbon, hydrogen and oxygen, with a variable side chain. Our body needs 20 different amino acids to synthesise all the proteins needed for growth as well as other metabolic functions. Of the 20 amino acids, nine are essential, meaning our body cannot synthesise them and must be taken in as food.

Atherosclerosis – discrete or patchy thickenings within the walls of arteries, called atherosclerotic plaques. If a plaque 'ruptures' it can cause blockage, and when this happens in arteries that supply blood to the heart (coronary arteries) it causes a heart attack.

ATP – Adenosine triphosphate is an organic compound which contains a large amount of chemical energy utilised by our cellular metabolic processes. ATP is produced by the mitochondria (powerhouse) of our cells by breaking down glucose.

Body mass index (BMI) – is a measure of our weight compared to our height and is a convenient way to broadly categorise a person as underweight, normal weight, overweight, or obese. For most adults the ideal BMI is in the 18.5 to 25 range.

CDC (Centers for Disease Control and Prevention) – a national public health institute in the United States. It is a US federal agency under the Department of Health and Human Services and is headquartered in Atlanta, Georgia. Its main goal is to protect public health and safety through the control and prevention of disease, injury and disability in the US and internationally.

Cholesterol – a chemical molecule belonging to the sterol group, a vital molecule found in every cell in the body. It is ubiquitous in the brain and essential for normal brain function, including learning and memory. Both the liver and the brain synthesise cholesterol; only 20 per cent of the cholesterol we need comes from our diet. High concentrations of cholesterol are found in egg yolks and seafood. It forms a part of many hormones including the sex hormones oestrogen and testosterone. It helps with the production of bile acids needed for digestion and is essential for the production of vitamin D, which is needed to maintain our bone structure. Cholesterol is essential – without it, we would die.

Clinical trial – a study method in which participants receive one or more drugs (medication) enabling researchers to evaluate the effect of these substances. When the study includes a group of patients who do not receive the treatment drug (the control group), it is called a 'controlled' trial.

Cytoplasm – all the material inside a cell, excluding the cell nucleus, and is enclosed by a cell membrane. It contains several organelles such as the mitochondria and is the site where most of the cellular chemical activities take place.

Disaccharide – the sugar formed when two simple sugars (monosaccharides) are joined together. Three common examples are sucrose (glucose + fructose), lactose (glucose + galactose) and maltose (glucose + glucose).

Double bond – a chemical term referring to the way two atoms are linked together. Fatty acid molecules with one or more double bonds are called unsaturated, while fatty acids without any double bonds are called saturated.

Fatty acids (fats) – consist of long chains of carbon and hydrogen atoms. When these substances combine with glycerol, fats are formed.

Genetic material – the most basic elements of genetic material are known as deoxyribonucleic acid (DNA) and ribonucleic acid (RNA). DNA is found in the nucleus of cells, while RNA is found in the cell cytoplasm. A gene consists of DNA molecules and is the basic unit of inheritance, which is passed from parents to their children. Genes determine our physical characteristics or traits. DNA is our genetic blueprint, while RNA is a copy of the blueprint, carrying the message of DNA and then 'translating' the message to form protein in the cytoplasm of the cell.

Genetic mutation – a gene mutation refers to a change or alteration that occurs in the DNA that forms a gene. Mutations range in size; they can affect a single DNA molecule or a large segment involving multiple genes. Mutations can be beneficial when it creates genetic diversity, keeping populations healthy but can also be harmful and result in disease. Many mutations have no effect at all and are called silent mutations.

Glycogen – the principal form in which glucose is stored in our muscle and liver tissue. Biochemically, it is a polysaccharide, with a branch-like structure. It can be utilised as an energy source when needed.

Insulin – a hormone produced by the pancreas which regulates blood glucose levels. It facilitates the movement of glucose from the blood stream into cells. It is also responsible for the storage of fat from extra glucose not utilised for energy and is, therefore, called the fat-storage hormone.

Macronutrient – the collective term used for carbohydrates, fats and proteins – the three food types that we consume in large quantities. Food is rarely solely composed of only one macronutrient, e.g. fats and proteins are found in meat, fish, eggs and dairy, while carbohydrates and proteins are found in vegetables, fruit, pulses and grains. A rare example of 100 per cent carbohydrate content is found in sugar while 100 per cent fat (monounsaturated) is found in olive oil.

Metabolism – an inclusive term, referring to all the breakdown biochemical reactions in the body, as well as reactions in which larger molecules are constructed from smaller ones.

Metabolic health – refers to a general healthy condition, with normal levels for all biomarkers – e.g. hormones such as insulin, and other blood biochemistry markers such as glucose, triglycerides etc. – without the use of medication.

Mitochondria – small structures (organelles) inside cells that produce energy (see ATP).

Monosaccharide – a simple sugar, the basic unit of carbohydrates. Examples include glucose, fructose and galactose. Monosaccharides are the building blocks of disaccharides.

Monounsaturated fats – fatty acids that contain a single double bond. This type of fat is most abundant in olive oil.

National Cholesterol Education Program (NCEP) – a programme managed by the National Heart, Lung and Blood Institute within the National Institutes of Health, US. It was created in 1985 to instruct Americans on how to avoid heart disease. It provides guidelines for doctors regarding ideal cholesterol levels and suggests treatment through lifestyle and drug (statin) therapy.

NHS (National Health Service) – the umbrella term for the publicly funded healthcare system of the United Kingdom (UK). It was established as one of the major social reforms following the Second World War in 1948 and is largely funded from general taxation.

Nucleus – an organelle within the cell where the DNA, containing all the genes, is situated. Genes control all the activities and functions of the cell and are, therefore, the control centre of the cell.

Osteoporosis – a condition that causes bones to become weak and brittle. It develops slowly over many years and is usually diagnosed when a fall or sudden impact causes a bone to fracture or break.

Pancreas – an organ in the abdomen that secretes enzymes responsible for the digestion of food and produces hormones such as insulin, which is important in glucose metabolism.

Phytoestrogens – plant-derived oestrogens (female hormones), also called the 'dietary oestrogens', because these compounds behave in a similar manner to natural oestrogen produced in the body. The highest concentrations are found in soybeans and soybean products followed by other members of the legume family. Several conditions and symptoms have been associated with the consumption of products containing phytoestrogens.

Polysaccharide – a carbohydrate molecule composed of multiple monosaccharide units, arranged in a chain-like pattern. For example, starch is a long chain of glucose molecules.

Polyunsaturated fats – fats in which the fatty acids contain two or more double bonds and are liquid at room temperature (oils). Omega-3 and omega-6 are both polyunsaturated fatty acids. Vegetable and seed oils are rich in omega-6.

Saturated fats (fatty acids) – a much-maligned category of fats. They generally range from 14 to 22 carbon atoms in length, with no double bonds. They are solid at room temperature (butter, tallow and lard) and predominantly found in food from animal sources.

Statins – a group of drugs that block the formation of cholesterol in the body. Statins reached the healthcare market first in 1987. They are sold on the premise that, by lowering cholesterol, they help prevent heart attacks and stroke. Their benefits are vastly overrated, e.g. for people not suffering from heart disease or without a history of a previous heart attack, taking a cholesterol-lowering statin pill will not prolong their life by one day. Statins are associated with serious side effects including increasing the risk of developing diabetes, Parkinson's and Alzheimer's disease, muscle and joint pains, fatigue, memory problems and heart failure to name a few.

Trans fat – industrially produced fat or fatty acid, where polyunsaturated oils are chemically further modified to be solid at room temperature. An example of such a product is margarine, now banned in many countries.

Unsaturated fat – a fat or fatty acid, containing one or more double bonds within the fatty acid carbon chain. These fatty acids are liquid at room temperature. The more double bonds in the fatty acid the more vulnerable it is to become rancid.

PERMISSIONS

Chapter 5 – Estimation of glycaemic loads: Dr David Unwin's NICE Endorsed Sugar Equivalence Infographics. This infographic is reproduced with permission from © Public Health Collaboration.

Chapter 7 – Food Industry Infographic: This infographic is reproduced with permission from © Oxfam America.

ABOUT THE AUTHORS

Estrelita van Rensburg

Trained as a medical doctor in South Africa, she specialised in virology and followed a research career as Professor and Head of Department at Stellenbosch University and the University of Pretoria for 16 years before joining the pharmaceutical industry in a global position. During this latter phase of her career, she became increasingly aware that the medical profession focused primarily on treating disease symptoms through prescribing medication, rather than finding preventative solutions.

Subsequently, when confronted with illnesses in family members and close friends, she further researched the area of preventative medicine. As part of her investigation, she discovered how misconceptions and misinformation regarding human nutrition, both in the mainstream media and the medical community, are important driving factors in the increase of modern-day lifestyle diseases.

With co-author Issy's help, they put together a healthy eating programme which showed amazing results, from both a health and body-weight perspective.

Issy Warrack

Issy comes from a real estate and business background, is a grandmother with two grandkids, always lived life to the full, and never gave her health a second thought. She never thought that ill health could happen to her until a series of events – heart palpitations and two falls resulting in fractures – happened. This was a real wake-up call. She knew she had to do something.

It was at that time that Estrelita started to research nutrition, and both decided that it was a no-brainer to seriously look at a healthy eating programme. It resulted in the Wellness EQ Programme, which made an immense difference to Issy. Her brain fog lifted, within weeks she lost weight, had more energy, her creative side returned, and she felt like a million dollars.

Printed in Great Britain
by Amazon